Fir ... Body Hoax

'A fant ... s a thoughtful view on a to ... for ourselves and our kid ... a very raw and hugely personal account of Emi's experience. Buy it and read it!'

'I enjoyed every page, it's passionate, funny and I have learnt an awful lot. I feel like I've had a few months of therapy!'

'A wonderfully honest, funny, but thought-provoking read about both a journey with cancer but more importantly our relationship with our own bodies.

Emi teaches us to value what is truly important and open our eyes to the 'lie' we have all been and continue to be, sold around body image.

Give this book to your children, both boys and girls, as they need our help now more than ever to see through this. We have one body, one life… love it and live it well.'

'It is a really good read and a fantastic topic to champion – one that completely resonates with me and which I think it is immensely helpful to have it written about.'

'Powerful, raw and thought-provoking.'

'I loved this book, I relate to so much of it.'

Dear Ruth ♡

THE BODY HOAX

How to Stop Believing in Fantasy Bodies

Emi Howe

Ditch the Glitch Wonderful human!

Emi x

Trigger Warning

Weights, body shape and size and BMIs will be mentioned in this book. This can be a trigger for those with eating disorders. Please bear this in mind before proceeding. If this or any of the other subjects in this book impact you, please refer to the support links at the back of the book.

First Printing, 2021
Circus Door Publishing

Contents

Dedication

For Mum
Thank you for my body

&

Liz and the NHS
Thank you for saving it

'Only those who attempt the absurd,
achieve the impossible.'

Albert Einstein

Prelude

Our great, great, great, great grandchildren:

'Did you know, in the Bronze Age, they believed the world was flat?'

'Just crazy! And in the Commercial Age, they believed that everyone could have a small, firm body!'
'Pah! Ridiculous!'

I Looked at it and Burst into Tears

About two years following my breast cancer diagnosis, I found a photo. It was a surgical photo of my headless, upper torso – these are taken for reference before and after each operation – this was the first one, taken before any surgery. I looked at it and burst into tears. My body was SO beautiful. How could I ever have thought that this body wasn't good enough? In that moment a realisation came into focus. I had been taught to feel like that. It wasn't real, but conditioned - programmed into me. I made it my mission to change The Glitch. I began to look at my body in different ways - less critical, less judgemental ways. I began searching for the ways my body supports me and thrives. The previous two years had provided me with a lot of good examples: its relentless march back to health after every toxin-filled chemo; its capability of giving and receiving love to my loved ones, to reassure them I'm OK *and* the ability to get out of bed to wash perfume out of my four-year-old's eye at 6.50 in the morning… with a chemo hangover! My body and its talents had been oppressed. And some new terms started floating to the surface for me: body loyalty; body pride; body respect; body love.

Over the following couple of years though, it became clear. It wasn't just *my* body that had been oppressed by a damaging cultural norm (The Glitch)… it was virtually everyone's. What must that mean, that level of widespread discontent? How does that impact us as individuals and as a society? I sought to find out, but what I found was worse than I had expected. We are living with A Glitch, a quiet one, that we don't pay attention to. It is taking our lives, either in small ways, by stealing our life's quality, or in big ways by stealing our life… altogether.

What's Your Body Shame?

For me it's my legs, specifically my calves. I know it's a bit random. Usually our body-shame focusses on belly, bum, even thighs, but calves? I have big, broad calves. In the past I have likened them to slabs of meat, to cankles (calf ankles with no distinction), like hams. They feel to me, out of proportion to the rest of my body. They are NOT feminine, beautiful, delicate, lithe or shapely; far from it. They are also not fat. (I will use the word fat as a descriptor throughout this book.) They are muscle. Strong, powerful, shotput-level muscle. So that's my body hang up, it's not a huge problem.

Yet, I have wasted *so much* of my life considering the rightness of my body. I look back on decades and wonder, what I could have done instead? The conversations I could have been having if I wasn't discussing my body, the places my thoughts could have lead me if I wasn't considering how to 'fix' my working-order body. The interests I could have developed, the skills I might have pursued. The world problems I might have contributed to solve, with all the other people who were not also sloshing out their life's potential with the body-bashing bathwater. What an absurd waste of our time, our lives! It is a loss and a potentially unnecessary one, because (I'm sorry to break it to you) our bodies may never change. And I'm not even the generation that's in the eye of the storm. Tweenagers ageing into the current landscape of bodies have an even harder job of snatching at reality, of knowing they are enough, of staying connected to themselves, when the world is telling them their value lies in staring into a camera, pout but for God's sake don't smile.

You may rightfully be wondering who I am and what I know about this? I'm a sociologist and a body therapist having delivered over 10,000 body therapies in my career. It has given me a good grasp of how we, as a society, feel about bodies, and it's not good news. Most clients apologise for their bodies, refer in jokey tones, to their unshaven legs, their fat, their inelegance or overdue hairdresser's appointment. I have no interest in anyone's body beyond how they feel inside of it, but it has been remarkably eye-opening to observe.

I'm also a breast cancer survivor of nine years, which gives me an insight into how we treat our bodies and how in turn, *they* treat us. Lastly I've grown up in a family that has been impacted by obesity. My Mum has been 'morbidly obese' (a misnomer) for my whole life. Along with Mum's blessing, we find out what that's like, as well as many other body differences. Ready for an adventure?

An Inconvenient Truth
This Crazy World

'This is the Eighties Mason, *nobody* likes reality anymore!'
Batteries Not Included – 1987

Post-Eighties, we have entered a period of astonishing standards of living. Smart phones and flat screen TVs are ubiquitous, even among the lowest income families. Grand Designs displaying ever-grander heights of living. The beautiful blogosphere advocating every health system under the sun: organic, vegan, lactose-free, keto, paleo, sugar-free. Prestige parenting - Kid Gods who dictate our existence – feed posts guilting us to get off our phones and parent already. A recent trend (even pre-Covid) of germ-phobia - unhealthy levels of cleanliness. So you see, it's not just bodies, they just form part of the impossible standards of modern living.

It's just all… too much. And none of it holds the self at the core - as important. It's others. Others' advice, others' values, others' directives that we collect like Pandora beads, others' opinions, standards, concepts, attention-grabbing, money-scoring, pressure-wielding impact. What it is not, is us connecting with ourselves, asking what WE need.

We've lost that connection.

We've become intolerant of feelings that aren't freaking blissful, or just happy, or even good! That's if we actually *feel* anymore at all and are not too busy taking a picture of the feeling, mentally writing an update about the feeling. We've attached visual provisos to feelings. How feelings should *look* - which further disconnects us from our experience of life. Intolerant of boredom, of imperfection or the reality that we're all different and performing differently on a myriad of scales. We all want the best of everything and we all believe there's a secret out there that will get it all for us. All of it. We want it all. Stuff, experiences, self-actualisation, credentials, prestige, status. We all want *all of the things* but what we don't realise is… we all have everything we actually need.

At the point of having everything we need, someone could have stepped in with some satisfaction training to teach people how to feel contented, to release dopamine. But what actually happened is we continued to search for needs and things to fulfil us, to attach meaning to – to release dopamine - so contentment was off the table. And so it goes on. False needs have been normalised in ever-more complex marketing portmanteaux: noseblindness, bedgasm, housebarassment – all words flitting around our current cultural landscape - all problems that aren't really problems beyond marketeers crowbarring them into our minds. When it should be easier, twenty-first century living is actually *more* stressful. While it's faster, more systematically efficient and intuitive, it is not more enlightened, kind, inclusive or healthy. It's not real. What we've gained rarely gets weighed up against what we've lost – it may look like progress but it's not as progressive as it seems. Maybe then the radical, rebellious, healthy act would be to stop trying to reach an unreachable (perpetually reinvented) height, but instead to unpick the fantasy and take a sigh of relief. Congratulations on being human, 0% robot.

But let's get back to bodies… Yes we have A Glitch, a kink in our reality, that has made us, well… miserable, self-critical. It limits us - it has stolen our quality of life. You'll know about The Glitch, because this is not new news - it's the (shrug) world we live in. The overused, exhaustive use of the 'ideal body' in our cultural landscape. It has been so normalised, we don't often identify it as separate from life. Our warped reality where thin bodies have been glorified, idealised, universalised, given top status. Thin/beauty ideals are used like a carrot to help us buy things we neither want or need. They are also used like a stick to beat us, in our minds and sometimes in our homes, schools, workplaces, doctor's surgeries and relationships. So not new news, check out the roll call of popular texts: *Fat is a Feminist Issue; The Beauty Myth; Reviving Ophelia; Body Positive Power; When Women Stop Hating Their Bodies; Body Talk; Body Gossip; Body Wars, The Truth about Fat, What We Don't Talk About When We Talk About Fat, Fattily Ever After, Just Eat It…*

We have known about the problem for decades, it impacts so many of us and yet the subject is still viewed as some kind of 'extreme feminism or aggression'.[1] Nothing has slowed down the steady cultural march further and further from reality with not even a tentative look back. You don't need me to point out that our media has washed itself of bodies that aren't thin, that fat shaming is still a prevalent and accepted form of discrimination, that 'fat talk' (the way we talk about ourselves and others in relation to weight) peppers our conversations and our thoughts. We harbour glitchy assumptions such as the rarely challenged 'weight loss is health' belief, the universal 'bad fat' rhetoric, the 'weight loss is for everyone' ruse – despite overwhelming evidence to the contrary. The idea that there is only one valid body. In self-development arenas these would be termed a 'limiting belief'. They limit us.

Yet still, it is *because* this stuff forms a big part of our core beliefs and how we understand the world, that it might smart to hear it. We've been conditioned to body dissatisfaction, most of us believe it's natural even. Just a part of us, that it can't be changed. It comes at a real loss to our lives, an unnecessary loss, one that we don't always notice because it's always been this way. In our culture of achievement, we have become a problem for the commercial world to fix.

So I'm not pointing that out.... But looking deeper and from different angles at The Glitch. To explain the cogs that keep it turning. It offers us an insight into the systems at play that keep this growing warped reality going and gives us the opportunity to decide if it's a direction we want to carry on in and if not, gives us some tools to help apply the brakes.

The Natural Diversity of Bodies

If you are wondering why you don't look like Nicole Kidman, Rihanna, Twiggy, Justin Bieber, Jamie Foxx, Jeff Goldblum, or any of those celebrities whose images bombard us each day, the answer is so simple. We are all different… and not photoshopped. We more readily accept that we are all different in almost every other aspect of our lives - celebrate it even. However, when it comes to bodies, we labour under the hokum that in just this one area, we must be, can surely all be, the same. Despite there being overwhelming evidence surrounding us every day in the shape of real people, living in our real world. I for one would hate that to change. I'd hate for our diversity to be lost and for us all to take on one figure or a very small range of figures, robotic, or lemming style. Perhaps you would too, but in holding that concept, does it bring up the thought – *it's fine for* other *people to be fat*? That's ok if it does, we've been trained to think like that. The media, especially the media of: health, fitness, wellbeing, self-care, diet culture, cosmetics, fashion, cosmetic surgery – these all repress, reject, deny and judge our natural diversity, with their own interests at heart.

Let's see how this actually works. Commenting in Psychology Today in 2010, Art Markham PhD introduces us to 'affected conditioning':

'One thing (adverts) do is to take a product and put it next to lots of other things that we already feel positively about. For example, an ad for detergent may have fresh flowers, cute babies, and sunshine in it. All of these are things that we probably feel pretty good about already. And repeatedly showing the detergent along with other things that we feel good about can make us feel good about the detergent, too. This transfer of our feelings from one set of items to another is called *affective conditioning* (the word affect means feelings).

'The feelings we have are often a good marker of what is safe to do and what is likely to turn out well. If we have to make a choice, and one of the options just feels good to us, then we are likely to go with the one that feels good.'[2]

What this means is that the world of advertising has leveraged this very human response and used it for their own gain. As Markham points out: 'They have paid for the opportunity to slip information to us about what feels good. That information ultimately affects the way we make choices, whether we know it or not.'[3]

This phenomenon has been proven to override even our knowledge of the product's properties. Researchers Dempsey and Mitchell completed a study assessing adverts, buying habits and choices, using pens. One brand of pen had clearly better properties. In the test group, the pen with worse properties was set against a series of positive images. Objectively the better pen should have been the one that the test group chose, and yet 70-80% of people exposed to the affective conditioning experiment, picked the inferior pen.[4] It should be noted by the way, that this phenomenon works best when we're not really paying attention to the advert at all.

Transfer the pen for a perfume and the feel-good image to a slender woman falling in love and repeat it, or a version of it, I don't know, a few hundred thousand times and you can see how, how we feel about our bodies and the connection we make of a thin body to positive outcomes has been conditioned in our minds.

We can also trace The Glitch back to the seventies and eighties. In 1980 Robert Crawford identified a shift towards what he called 'healthism' or the 'Medicalisation of Everyday Life'[5]. It was the rise of the fitness boom with the launch of many health and fitness magazines, the steep interest in aerobics and fitness classes, shows and videos, workout celebrities greeting us through our screens at breakfast. It has never really occurred to me before (and why would it, this shift happened before I was born) that how we view health hasn't always been like this. Something had changed. The business of our health had morphed from being the concern of our doctors, to being placed firmly on *our* shoulders. Health *and* adverse health was now our fault. We were now much more active in the process. Good health needed a clear vision, a marker, a standard… and it was thin. I mean, thinness was coveted before then, it just wasn't so heavily placed in our laps, and it was so much easier to convey as a health marker than cholesterol or blood pressure stats, sexier too! Sexy, and too simplistic.

The Glitch is a problem without an adequate solution and has manifested in a loss of connection with our bodies and the undermining of our health and more. Lemmings is a bit strong of a word though, isn't it? It smacks of brain-washing, of sheep, of glazed-eyed ghouls with no independent direction…

We have a way of talking about bodies that assumes thinness is for everyone. It is based on the very basics of how a body works – it's kindergarten stuff.

Move more + eat less = be thin.

For many people their body intelligence / awareness stops there, when in fact there's an awful lot more knowledge we need, to truly understand our bodies. Body image thought leader, Jean Kilbourn in her 1995 Documentary *Slim Hopes* identifies that the ideal body is naturally achievable for less than 5% of women[6]. If facial features and such are to be taken into account that figure drops to more like 1%[7,8] - a fantasy body for 99% of the population. That magical silhouette we're attempting to achieve or any attribute of it, is actually more of a quirk of nature - one that in its very selection for the job (usually model, also presenter, movie or music star), has been filtered so heavily away from many thousands of other bodies and presented as to appear common, that we have come to believe in it. It ISN'T real. Your 'dream body' is a well-marketed anomaly. It doesn't exist in most of us. You can't diet into it.

What's more, we never see abstract bodies the way we most frequently see our own – putting on our socks, going to the loo, getting in the bath, during sex. Times that give us pause, to consider the rightness of our bodies under vastly incomparable conditions. We've assigned false beliefs to our: food, clothes, bodies and in doing so we've created more work for ourselves – turned ourselves into a job.

As we have, for the most part, grown up with The Glitch and may not have noticed it, it has been a background conversation of unchecked diet culture, where thin is perceived as: healthy, good, successful, sexy, valid. And all other bodies are not. We may not have noticed how we pay more attention to our bodies than almost anything else. In 2007, sociologist and researcher Christie Newman wrote about the advent of a dubious 'healthy femininity' as being 'committed to the pursuit of health, longevity and wellbeing above all other concerns'[9]. Another study discovered that 63% of us view weight as the main factor influencing how we feel about ourselves above family, school or work[10].

Our lives have been commercialised to such a degree and we often now only view them through that filter, that bias has been programmed into us. As such, we have lost touch with ourselves and our relationship with our bodies. With what *we* actually want, are interested in, can afford. Maybe lemmings IS the right word after all. Let's be honest, we don't often stop to catch ourselves and think – *that was a commercially-driven thought.*

In fact what we actually want is so deeply buried we may not even know it's there! We relate to our bodies in terms of how they relate to other things – clothes, food, men, women, friends, status, not how it feels to live in them when arguably that is the thing that most directly impacts us. What they provide, how they support us, how efficient they are and evolved to survive. How it feels to live in them. They are one highly specific piece of kit, with millions of working parts!

Anyway, because I'm keen to live in the real world after all and I'm eager to recognise, accept and champion the natural diversity of bodies, it demands that I accept *my role* in the natural diversity of bodies, mega-calves and all. As you can see, from the cover of this book, I am fairly slim. So maybe you're wondering what I have to moan about? Simply, it's because it's all the women – well, over 90% of us – who are dissatisfied with our bodies – who are jettisoning our feel-good in favour of self-criticism - and that's too many. And it's not just women, men, trans and non-binary people report increased feelings of body dissatisfaction too. It's actually fairly messed up – especially as it's a fabricated and overly simplified problem. And although my experience of The Glitch, I feel, has been life-limiting – a loss of my quality of life (unnecessary loss), through tiny pin-pricks of self-esteem seeping out of me, my experience is *nothing*. Nothing compared to those who live in marginalised bodies. For true fat education (and we do all need it) please head over to Aubrey Gordon's book *What We Don't Talk About When We Talk About Fat* [11] and Stephanie Yeboah's *Fattily Ever After* [12] to really discover what that lived experience is. I can't speak to that, but *they* can and they do it well.

So a problem where ALL bodies have been condemned. Newman's 2007 work features the anecdotal comment: 'If you are plump, you are teased. If you are thin, certain women become bitchy.'[13] There are cultural narratives to draw anxiety out of people with every type of body.

Beyond this being just about learning to accept our place in the natural diversity of bodies, there is something more sinister at play. The Glitch is making people… fat and it's a fine balance here because I am definitely advocating that fat bodies are valid, vital, healthy (you'll see), beautiful, valuable, sexy, equal. While holding in my other hand a magnifying glass focussed on a cultural worm that is insidiously making us put on weight, that some of us might want to learn more about.

Yes, our narrative, our beliefs, our commentary and conversations are often *contributing* to the one thing they're trying to banish - fatness. There is a sad irony that the hysteria around the 'obesity crisis' is contributing to… the 'obesity crisis'. If this seems implausible, don't worry, there's a whole chapter on this coming up. With that in mind, let's talk about how this book is going to take shape.

We're going to take a potted history lesson of bodies in a section called *Conversations That* Probably *Never Happened.*

We're going to further explore body connection by looking at how my relationship with my body has been shaped, some of it you might recognise from your own past, and other bits you might not (bye bye nipples) We're then going to dive deep into the reality of bodies. What makes us the glorious, diverse society that we are - truth-seekers most welcome. We're then going to pick apart the way that we're unwittingly making ourselves fatter. We'll also look at inclusion and how to become an ally.

Nearing the end, I'm going to introduce you to the campaign I headed up asking for better representation of bodies in advertising and look to our establishment. I'm going to share with you the answers to questions I've had for decades about why we feel the way we do.

Throughout the book, look out for Body Stories. Where I ask others to share their views. Real people from all walks of life, sharing intimate body thoughts that just don't often get aired. We talk about ideals, thinness and fantasy bodies much more than our actual realness!

I want every person to have this knowledge in their brains. Knowledge about the systems at play that make us feel the way we do about our real bodies. All while trying as best I can, not to throw anyone under the bus. Because you cannot know what you do not know. We are products of our own making here in this problem. All of us have grown up in and have been influenced by and *even* contributed to the *fantasy world of thin* - where thinness feels as right as oxygen and so far there haven't been enough interventions to correct that. *The Body Hoax helps* us to see how appropriate it would be to Value Real Bodies, on a mainstream, cultural level. The question is, how do we elevate this subject into that place? I've got a couple of good ideas… But first let's get back to:

Our Great, Great, Great, Great Grandchildren:

'Did you know, in the Bronze Age, they believed the world was flat?'

'Just crazy! *And* in the Commercial Age, they thought that everyone could have a small-firm body!'

'Pah! Ridiculous. Why did it take them so long to figure out that we all have different bodies?'

'Hang on, I know this one, I read it somewhere, let me just… ah yes, here it is. It was something called… diet culture and the thin/beauty ideal.'

'Diet?'

'Yes, it was a theory of eating less food and exercising more, as a means to determine their bodies.'

'Right. Did it work?'

'Ha, hell no! They were usually phenomenally unsuccessful.'

'So why did they keep doing it?'

'A lot of reasons but ultimately, it seems, they didn't want to stop believing it would work.'

'Believe what would work?'

'That they'd make a small-firm body.'

'What's so good about a small-firm body?'

'I know right? But in those times, a lot of false meanings were attached to having one, partly because almost *all* of the best image jobs went to small-firm-bodied people. Remember they were *ruled* by image back then; and bear in mind, this was before the Equality Amnesty or the True Wellbeing Revolution. Such different times. It was based on out-dated science blended with mythology and folklore that flooded the whole society. It kept continually being reinforced so that before long, the society itself was growing the ruse, thinking it was true. Content creators believed it, government believed it, parents believed it, doctors believed it, everyone did!'

'Even though they MUST have been surrounded by real bodies of all different shapes and sizes?'

'There were *even more* extremes of sizes back then, but yes the belief that everyone could and should be small-firm, was strong. You can't blame them, it was a pretty convincing racket. So much so, it wasn't seen as a theory, but more accepted as truth, science… law, even though SO MANY academic papers of that time disproved it, nobody seemed to pay any attention. And I think the reason is that diet culture made some people very, very rich.'

'A product not working, made some people very *rich*?'

'It not only didn't work, in many cases it had the *opposite* effect. Causing many people, say, with naturally medium bodies to do diet culture and actually get big-soft ones in the long run, which because they worshipped small-firm ones instead, made them want to start the diet culture all over again! And as for the academics disproving the point, THEY had nothing to sell, the commercial world overwhelmingly drowned them out and kept diverting attention back to diet culture and small-firm bodies.'

'I don't believe you. That's fiction!'

'I tell you, it's the truth!'

The Birth of the Beauty Industry

Conversations that *Probably* Never Happened

3 Million BC, Bedrock

Wilma: Betty, what are you doing?

Betty: Oh I'm just trying something out.

Betty has a clamshell pursed between her finger and thumb. Whatever she's doing is causing her to yelp intermittently. On closer inspection, Wilma finds that Betty is using the shell to pull out the hairs around her ankles.

Wilma: Betty! For the love of Lionhide, what are you doing?

Betty: I'm getting rid of these hairs.

Wilma: Whatever for? Have you gone mad? *And* Winter's coming!

Betty (silent for some time and looking stricken): Barney has strayed Wilma. I've seen him looking longingly at The Bonespear Girl. All young and fair. And look at me! I *have* to do something!

Wilma: Barney? Are you sure?

Betty: I sure am! I caught them, laughing like cave-children while they were scraping the bison hide yesterday. He said (Betty stops and lets out a sob) 'This feels like Betty's legs'!

Wilma: Oh Betty.

Betty: And that Bonespear Girl only went and put out one of her own fair-haired legs in comparison!

Wilma: But Barney…

Betty: And he… *stroked* her leg Wilma! Practically went cross-eyed with joy!

Wilma: Do you know, Fred would have done the exact same thing. I don't think he will have meant any…

Betty: And then! Then she was collecting water down at Watery Hole, Barney was passing on his way out to hunt the warthogs. I saw her jump into the water and call out to him, splashing her long legs out of the water.

Wilma: And what did he say?

Betty: I don't know, I couldn't hear.

The women sat in silence, pierced only by Betty's continued yelping. Eventually…

Wilma: Do you think it has anything to do with Mr Bonespear being gone these five years?

Suddenly the BoneSpear Girl appears.

Bonespear Girl: Hey what's that!

Betty (glowering): It's a… shell.

Bonespear Girl: But what are you doing with it?

Betty: Nothing.

Wilma: It's a pelt tamer.

Bonespear Girl: Wow! A pelt tamer. Can I get one? Where can I get one?

Wilma: Oh they're very rare. Maybe you could have this one.

Betty: Hey!

Wilma (with a knowing look to Betty): Just five hides and it's yours.

The Bonespear Girl, gave it some thought before agreeing. She skipped off with her Pelt Tamer.

Betty: What you go and do that for?

Wilma: Because you're going to need something to cover up those bald ankles… and anyway, I can't sit and listen to you *yelp* any more!

The Birth of Influencers and the Selfie

Conversations that *Probably* Never Happened
A London Shack in the Middle Ages.

Inside, sisters are doing their toilet. Agnes is applying a white substance to her face. Isabella is lying down with bandages draping her forehead and hairline.

Agnes: 'Ere, what d'you reckon about the end of Queen Liz then?
Isabella: Well, down the market they reckon she was a right sight! Ravin' like a mad woman! Did you 'ere?
Agnes: 'Ere what?
Isabella: Well Ralph the Veg Man, says Walter the Barrow Boy, spoke wiv William the Maker of Spice Bags for the palace, he 'eard from Beatrice, the Lady o' the Bed Chamber, reckons it was *poison* of the blood.
Agnes: Like murder?
Isabella: No, I dunno. In any case, she refused to let anyone look at 'er body so I s'pose we'll never know.
Agnes: Well, if nofink else, she left us beauty, taught all us how to be elegant and refined. What a bunch of old hags we'd be if not for her.
The sisters smiled, bearing missing teeth.
Isabella: I 'eard a rumour from Mrs Fritz down the river.
Agnes: Oh yeah, what's that ol' trout got to say?
Isabella: She reckons it was the Venetian Ceruse.
Agnes: What? This? Agnes motioned to the white substance in her hand.

Isabella: Not that you silly goose. That's made out of ash and eggs! No, the posh stuff, like what the toffs wear. Said *it* was the poison and get this, get this!
Agnes: What!
Isabella: Mrs Fritz reckons that Venetian Ceruse rotted Queenie's hair away!
Agnes: *Rotted* it away? Ha I *don't* think so. Look at you! Lying there, bandages soaked in cat piss on yer 'ead. I don't think you'd be doing that to get rid of *your* hair would ya! If it were 'cause someone's hair rotted off. Don't be daft!
Isabella: Well exactly, and how else are we ladies meant to make a livin' off them toffs, if we look like any ol' common muck? Elegant, we are.
Agnes and Isabella laughed in unison.
Agnes: Tell you what though.
Isabella: What's that?
Agnes: It'd be nice not having to chase those flippin' cats around all day!
They nodded in contemplative silence.

Queen Elizabeth I, contracted small pox at the age of 29, it left her with scars and she used the heavy white makeup made out of white lead and vinegar, to cover them – her 'mask' to keep her looking youthful. However it also initiated a trend among women of white faces, removal of eyebrows and the hairline and lavish wigs. She died at age 69 of possible blood poisoning.

Venetian Ceruse was classified as poisonous 31 years after Queen Elizabeth I's death. Reports of the end of her life had her wearing a full inch of the make-up on her face, having lost most of her teeth, hair, and she wouldn't be attended to or bathed. G. J. Meyers describes her as 'a pathetic spectacle, all the more so because throughout her reign she had been vain to the point of childishness.'[14, 15]

Artist Mat Collishaw has made a mask that tried to reveal the truth of Queen Elizabeth I's actual appearance has this to say:

'Propaganda portraiture was once the reserve of the rich and powerful but it's now in the hands of every teenager: the ability to curate your image to present a persona to the world. This ability is empowering but also quite perilous, as it's easy to develop the addiction to presenting a positive image of yourself, far from reality, to mask vulnerability and insecurity. Elizabeth pioneered this syndrome.'[16]

The Birth of Body Sculpting

Conversations that *Probably* Never Happened

Green Park Ladies College 1860s

Dear Mama,

I have arrived, made my safe arrival at Green Park, all is well though the journey arduous.

I have met one friend already, Matilda, her family hail from the country too. The food has been rather light, only a few leaves so far. I'm hoping for a more robust meal later this evening. Oh how I shall miss Cook's pot pies and jam puffs!

One thing I am surprised by is the issue of a new corset. The headmistress, Ms Shuttleworth was clear in her instructions and I was laced into it almost on arrival. Never in my life have I experienced such tight lacing Mama, and I really don't know how I shall bear it! I can barely breathe! Matilda assures me I shall get used to it. It was only then that I noticed her waist. I could practically fit my hands around it! I am *most* perturbed.

My room is cold but clean enough and unpacking was no great chore. Gosh I do hope they call us for dinner soon, I'm famished!

I shall write again soon Mama, missing you all.

Audrey

Dear Mama,

I write in plea, mother, please send a carriage or if nothing else some sustenance. Cook's shortbreads or a turnover at the very least! I cannot stay these conditions. Since my last letter, I have been perpetually in my corset, morning, noon *and* night! The only time it has been manoeuvred is to tighten it still! At a point that I could no longer breathe and only panic could rise from me. I haven't had a proper meal and instead am fed on scraps of greenery.

Matilda keeps trying to convince me I will absorb this new habit, if I can bear the pain, she says, it will pass in a while, but I'm sure I won't adjust. Oh to breathe! The other girls seem to be in some sort of wonderland of perverse reality, where this corset tightening is something of pride, of elation even! It's as if their brains have been washed of their senses! I am aware this schooling is all in my best interests but I really think my piano-playing will suffice in capturing the admiring glances of a decent man. Mr Foxpatrick himself offered his congratulations after my last recital! Mother please send for me!

Yours in desperation,

Audrey

Mama,

Are my letters not reaching you? I have reached the end of my first month here at Green Park and really feel that Jane could be imparting these lessons. Never a better Governess there was.

You may wonder how I'm fairing with my corset. I have had it removed for the time of just one hour per week since my arrival, this is designed as bathing time but is nothing short of torture. My skin itches like the pox and is red and unsightly. I could claw it off and any form of ablution feels like nettle stings! The corset, measured before and after, will always be tightened to measure the same or *even* smaller! I am finding it virtually impossible to sleep, to eat, to take leisure. Oh to snack on jellied pineapple, marrow toast! Or heaven grant me, a pressed duck!

I would rather live with Aunt Beaumount than spend another minute in this dungeon!

Please send the carriage!
I'm begging.
Audrey

The Estate of Lord and Lady Pinningbury

Mama: Audrey! How lovely it is to have you at home with the family. And just look! The image of modern refinement! I'm so sorry I couldn't be at your finishing ceremony from Green Park but Ms Shuttleworth tells me you passed with flying colours: needlepoint, flower-arranging and a thirteen inch waist to boot!
Audrey: I expect nothing less Mother as you haven't replied to my letters for such a time. You missed nothing, I fainted at the ceremony, it was a huge embarrassment.
Mama: Audrey I know you feel badly about the corset. It's simply a right of passage, a sacrifice we all must make, in securing our future, our estate even! And look at you! The picture of status and beauty. Your shoulder blades, why I even think they're touching. You did it for the family and we thank you.
Audrey eyeballed Mama's expansive waistline.
Mama: Speaking of… we have an invitation from the Foxpatricks this *very* evening, so we better smarten ourselves up! Chop chop!

Post script: In her book *How to be a Victorian*, Ruth Goodman calls this: 'The age of the corset horror story' with corsets impacting: breathing, voice, digestion, reproduction and the deformation of the skeleton.

'To put this into perspective, the waist measurement of the average toddler is about twenty inches. Such drastic reductions in waist size could be achieved only by a women wearing, over a period of time, a series of smaller and smaller garments and corsets, both day and night, and eating a very regulated diet with a number of tiny meals replacing the three main meals of the day.'[17]

The Birth of the Model

Conversations that *Probably* Never Happened
Battle Creek, Michigan – circa 1927

'Heathen!'

'What troubles you Brother?' Will Kellogg took off his wire-rimmed glasses.

'That scoundrel Ernest Bernays and his Freudian quackery, has stolen *my* phrase. This newspaper says he is claiming breakfast as being the "The most important meal of the day!" *He* doesn't claim it, *I* do!' John adjusted his white tie, in his tight white collar. 'Breakfast is *cereal*, do you know what he is claiming that breakfast should be?'

John's wife Ella, absent-mindedly adjusted a tapestry on the parlour wall, it bears the words 'My soul finds rest in God alone'.

'What's that dear?'

'Bacon! Of all things. *Bacon*! Don't they realise what meat does to a person?'

'Most don't my love' Ella sighed wistfully, 'the sexual urges, the inappropriate touching. The world will learn, in the fullness of time,' her voice changed key, 'the failures of the flesh.' As she talked, she shooed out one of her many adopted children (her marriage never having been consummated).

Will, the younger, more considered and less ostentatious of the two brothers remarked, 'I read a book by that Bernays chap, called *Propaganda*. It made for quite an interesting read, let me find it. John folded his arms across his lily-white suit lapels and coughed. Will found the marked page and began to read aloud:

'The conscious and intelligent manipulation of the organized habits and opinions of the masses is an important element in democratic society. Those who manipulate this unseen mechanism of society constitute an invisible government which is the true ruling power of our country. We are governed, our minds are moulded, our tastes formed, and our ideas suggested, largely by men we have never heard of.... It is they who pull the wires that control the public mind.' 18

Will continued - 'He talks of ways to control the populace, without them even *knowing* it, not by reason, but by making them *feel* things! He has proved it quite powerful - in his work for the war effort, helping recruit all those boys.'

Will's wife Carrie looked up from her needlepoint and joined the conversation with uncertainty. 'Isn't he the man that encouraged women to start smoking cigarettes? Called them "Torches of Freedom". Can't be healthy. Most questionable morality, surely darling, only greed'.

'But of course, dear, we could use the same principles for good? Change the habits of the masses, help them to engage in *healthier* practices. By replacing bacon with... our cereal for example,' Will sat back and removed his tiny rosette necktie. Molly the parlour maid arrived carrying refreshments.

John uncrossed his sugar-white-trousered legs and leaned in. 'By what means brother?'

'Well, we have had significant success with the advertisement these twenty-five years', he explained, 'I have taken the liberty to stage a new idea.'

A paper exchanged between the two men. John opened it up and falteringly read it aloud.

'"I've got to feel my best, to *look* my best." Joan Hoff, well-known photographer's model "That's why I'm strong for the self-starter breakfast."'[19]

Carrie wrinkled her nose. 'I'm sure I don't understand. What does a photographer's model have to do with breakfast cereal?'

John continued to consider the advertisement from different angles. 'Well I can see... how...' he passed it to Carrie. Her eyes widened.

'She's *very* glamourous. She stared at the picture for some time. Her thoughts unclear. Eventually she said 'I'm not sure what I have in common with her though, why it would make me want to buy cereal. Anyway, wouldn't it be much better for people to see versions of themselves? This glamour is too far removed'. The fire licked and curled in the grate.

'But that's exactly the point I'm guessing.' John eased his cotton-white-socked feet out of his snowy brogues. 'You *aren't* her; you want to *be* her. It makes you *feel* something.' Carrie considered the print again. Her look of bafflement rising to surprise in realisation; then crumpling back to quizzical.

'But how is a breakfast cereal going to make *me*, like *her*?' she asked, looking first at her husband and then at John.

'The point Bernays is trying to make darling,' Will explained, unsmiling as ever, 'is that... it doesn't really matter.'

'And if it works,' John slapped Will on the back 'then we have a way of making these sinful meat-chompers healthy again!' The brothers slurped at their cups contentedly in self-congratulation.

'But, if I'm not mistaken, you're proposing to make, women particularly, feel like they're missing something... and not fill in the gap? Is that fair? I'm just not sure it's right... is it?'

A look crossed between the brethren. Ella announced 'Carrie be a dear and close the drapes, I can feel a chill coming in.' Will seemed troubled 'Can you say what is taken away exactly? From women?' Carrie considered this, gazing out into the deep night. 'Um, I, well… I can't quite…'

If she'd listened carefully, she would have heard the whispers of a thousand women through the decades on the wind: 'Your enoughness'. But she'd already closed the drapes.

'Propaganda you call it?' John asked of Will.

'That's right, although I think it is also known now as "Public Relations."'

Postscript: The Bernays' Beech Nut Bacon stunt happened in 1920's and the cereal ad ran in 1931.[20] It was a time for a new era of ideas around manipulation in advertising. The run-away success of Edward Bernays' smoking campaign for Lucky Strike, where he inspired women to use smoking as a tool for empowerment, earned him accolades of both PR Guru and mass murderer posthumously.

The Birth of Photoshop

Conversations that Probably Never Happened

Ann Arbor, Michigan, USA 1987

John: I don't think you realise what you've just invented bro!

Thomas: Yeah! It's exciting! It's not going to get my PhD done though!

John: I… think this is going to be bigger than that. I mean this is going to *revolutionise* the movie industry, architecture, publishing…

Thomas: I'm just enjoying messing around with these photos I took over the creek, how you can play with the light. And look, this kingfisher is taken from a completely different picture!

John: Yeah, the scope is… almost infinite. Does it have a name?

Thomas: I thought, Image Pro…

The brothers are working away in companiable silence while they consider the name.

John: Check it out!

Thomas comes to look at John's monitor. On it is the world's first official photoshopped image. It is of a paradise island and in the foreground, a topless woman with her back to us.

Thomas: What's the woman got to do with it?

John (shrugs): Adds interest, otherwise it's just a picture of the sea! I call it, *Jennifer in Paradise.*[21]

Days later…

John: Turns out 'Image Pro' is already being used.

Thomas: What about… Photo Lab?

John: That might work…

Thomas: John?

John: Yeah?

Thomas: Do you think we need to consider testing the product.

John: Oh yeah, the studio are on board for trying it out. And market research will have to be done.

Thomas: No I mean, I've created this product that edits and manipulates images. It sort of… warps reality. Do we have a duty to see what the long-term effects of that might have, you know on people using it, seeing the end results?

John (giving it a lot of thought): But this is tech, not medicine! I mean, if you want it to take years to get into production and give someone else the chance to get it out there first!

Thomas: Yeah, it would kind of derail the project.

John: Especially if the answer is yes! Also, bro, you're clever but you're going to shift what? Like at most 500 units a month? It's not like you're going to shape the way people look at the world to the point that we *live in a warped reality!*

John throws a balled piece of paper at Thomas who laughs and ducks out of the way.

Postscript: This conversation is obviously a fabrication - I have no idea if this concept was even on the table in 1987, I was eight years old. I know that concepts such as wellness, mental health, the impact of idealised living, corporate wellbeing were not the subjects that they are today. A person cannot know what they don't know. Before the product was created, I imagine it would have been very hard to foresee its drawbacks. Such a ground-breaking technology couldn't have, wouldn't have been shelved on the grounds that *maybe* the long-term effects might not be great. Despite our obsession with health and wellbeing, they're not important enough to stand in the way of progress. In addition we have a case of diffused responsibility, where image manipulation of a kind did already exist and since then, every individual who has ever used photoshop to enhance and manipulate an image, every editor who has asked for it or signed it off, is culpable for our current visual landscape of unreality and *is* going forwards. Photoshop has some really cool features, and if used responsibly can enhance our world. If not for photoshop, the front cover of this book wouldn't be what it is!

Responsible use would include: not idealising / perfecting images to the point of unreality; thereby not setting unreachable, impossible standards; if that does have to happen, including some sort of label to make the fakery explicit… as a matter of public health.

In fact, Photoshop sold to Adobe eight years later for $34.5 million. In 2019 the brothers were honoured at the Oscars with the *Scientific and Engineering Award* for the original architecture, design and development of *Photoshop.*

Thomas has this to say: 'It turned out really well. One of the times that I realise the influence this little project has had on the world, is when watching a TV show or a movie and they actually use photoshop as a verb. I know Adobe legal doesn't like that because of the use of trademarks, but it gives me a little thrill every time I hear that. It's quite neat to have a verb that you created.'[22], [23]

'Photoshop' must have different connotations for him, than it does for me…

'Definition of *photoshop*

transitive verb

:to alter (a digital image) with *Photoshop* software or other image-editing software especially in a way that distorts reality (as for deliberately deceptive purposes)'[24]

My Body, My Life

Age Four

'But you *PROMISED*!' I screamed with the outrage only a spurned four-year-old can muster. Sitting on the Formica kitchen worktop, grubby legs hanging, Mummy and Daddy askance.

'No, I said it *might* need stitches.'

'I want *stitches*!'

'Over the phone I can't have known what it would need, I hadn't even *seen* it Pet!'

Earlier, I'd stared at my reflection in a head-height brass letterbox, tributaries of blood covering my face. There had been a Bluebird bike – training wheels recently jettisoned - a bollard, quick-working brakes, the smell of fresh tarmac on a new path… and an eyebrow.

Daddy (a doctor) ventured 'Sometimes, instead of a stitch, the doctor uses these Steristrips. They're much better actually as they don't hurt as much. For a smaller cut like this, they'll be fine.'

'It's *not* small!' I remonstrated…

I knew my body and how I wanted it used - as a tool, for new experiences, that require an adventure, to a hospital and the gleeful repercussions of attention and general showoffery. I had no concept that, that day would live in every mirror I'd look in, for the rest of my life, because I only viewed my body as myself.

Age Seven

This was around the time that I realised my Mum wasn't like other Mums. She was fat. Non-active. I am ashamed of the shame I felt about this. She is also acutely afraid of swimming; I love swimming.

I don't remember feeling disappointment that she was unable to do many active things with me. It just was. But I didn't understand it and nobody could explain it to me.

Age 15

Lazing in the hammock in next-door's garden. It's 1994. The soundtrack of the summer was Dawn Penn's *No no no no*, Crash Test Dummies' *Mmm mmm mmm mmm* and Doop's *Doop doop doop doop do do do.* It was stirring stuff.

I was reading a magazine, absorbing the bodies. 90's Teen magazines, the Mizzes, Just 17s, more!s and they were basically just bodies - as if a teenage girl has nothing more stimulating to think about. But in the summer the bodies got browner, bronzer, sandier, nakeder, tousleder, wrapped in tropical bikinis, doused in Hawaiian Tropic, sipping hypercolour cocktails and *prescriptive.* It all gets very directive, for how you too, dear reader, not only can but *should* achieve such greatness. For starters, scrubbing, brushing, rubbing, kneading, depilating.

File those hooves down, rub them too, while you're there. *All* the time. And cleanse, tone and moisturise and for God's sake shave woman! *Or* wax or bleach or cut or epilate. Flippin' 'eck! Where was I going to find the time? Or the money for all of this? At fifteen?

Money. Because it's all about money. It is *only* about money. *Doll it was never about you.* (It's worth noting at this stage in the book how many times money is going to come up in this conversation.)

But on this particular day I was reading something even more sinister. An article prescribing the circumference of the 'perfect' legs. Yep, three measurements to fixate on. And gaps, where they should be, between my legs, for them to be… *right.* I mean also I had *real* problems like trying not to fart in assembly or burn down my bedroom with cheap candles.

And that was it. That was the moment that my connection with my body broke.

Did you know a muscle is like a rope and when you injure it, it's usually because some of the fibres of the rope have snapped. I visualise my body connection now like a muscle and although splitting will have occurred before this, a significant bunch of them ripped now.

Of course, no teenager is a blank canvas, I knew the BS going on and the weird duality of this unreal system. Would belly-ache about it with my friends. They entertained it but most of them were just like 'whatever'. What could I do about it? I concluded, nothing.

Yet of course I still roused myself from the hammock a different person. Two people actually. Myself as I always had been and a new version with a firm appreciation for how *others* viewed me - I didn't know that at the time of course. We both headed through the neighbour's house, onto the path, into my house, into the dining room, into the rattan basket under the stacked stereo turntable to find my Mum's sewing kit and tape measure. Just as I expected with my mega calves… *inches* out. It was official, my legs were wrong! It would be another 20 years before my legs were right again and I started knitting my two sides back together.

What a mind-boggling waste, astonishing really. And it wasn't the worst, people have worse problems, but just everything, every joyful experience being tainted by a not-good-enough thought-backdrop. It's criminal. A health crime! How much feel-good was sacrificed, lost, frittered in the name of fakery and nonsense? And at what cost… to me? Who might I have been, had I not been fixated with my body? And throughout it all, was I unhealthy? (I mean growing cancer aside) No, I never veered into an unhealthy BMI – whatever that means. I just didn't conform to the idealised body and felt variously shame, frustration, sadness, unworthiness, anxiety, just not any good. All classic hallmarks of stress. All not healthy. I want you to also look out in this book, for references of people spending their lives 'proving my worth', and be conscious of the energy and effort that goes into that. If trying to do such a thing is even possible, based on other people's appraisal of us or a fabricated ideal.

But I did try to conform with the scrubbing and the rubbing and the dieting and the running and the shaving of course. But then in real life, I moved on to college and discovered alcohol, I moved on to university and had to make my own food! All the while conforming to the unspoken sisterhood code of 'we must hate our bodies'. I would disrespect it, talk badly about it, dismiss it and objectify it, and that helped me fit in, because what kind of shmuck likes their body?

At this point, I want to look at some other women's coming of age stories…

Body Stories
Georgie

I come from a family that don't 'do' affection or praise. I remember my Mum walking me to school one day and talking about all the girls in my class and how pretty they were. I asked her if she thought I was pretty and her reply affects me to this day, 'You're not pretty, but you're attractive'. I know what she meant now, but to an 11-year-old she might as well have told me I was pig ugly.

It's only in adulthood, and having become a parent myself, that I realise how important it is to feel loved and to be praised and in spite of my experience, I have become a better parent and know what not to do to provide your children with the building blocks they need to love themselves and to have a positive image of themselves, as well as putting themselves in the shoes of others before they judge.

I've never had much self-esteem and whatever I have had, I've created myself from wearing make-up, buying clothes etc. This self-built esteem doesn't seem to have strong foundations and is absolutely flattened by the smallest of things including criticism which has carried through to my adulthood and even now, affects my relationships - I married a physical and mental bully - and into my work life.

Things went downhill when my parents divorced. Not only did I lose my home, I lost my school friends and moved three hours away from my Dad. I was 11, and the following years leading to my teens were affected by my mother who, having been badly impacted by my father's infidelity, made the most awful life choices (involving men and drinking unfortunately, not what was best for her kids).

I moved schools too many times to remember and always being the new kid with ginger hair and a posh accent meant I was bullied profoundly. The worst was when I moved to a really rough school near Liverpool, I got groped constantly, thrown down stairs, my hair pulled out in clumps, spat at and throttled so hard I almost passed out. I walked the five miles home quite often to get some relief. That period of time instilled the worthless factor in me for a very long time, and still does to some extent. I was always looking at other girls, wishing I was prettier, thinner, not ginger etc. and all the while, my 'safety net' at home gave me no tools to help me fight this. I attempted to cut my wrists on more than one occasion.

As an adult I have learnt to look at these experiences positively and in some ways it's made me a more determined person, I do things I never thought I would. I've done triathlons, long distance open water swims, run 10ks, jumped out of planes and worked hard in my career. All of these things make my self-image slightly more positive as I know my bullies and my parents haven't done any of these things so I've proved myself. I am also a better parent because of it. I ensure my son gets the affection and attention he needs, we talk openly about the way he sees himself and others, as well as knowing how to recognise all forms of bullying and to talk about it if he needs to.

Self-image isn't just a physical concept, it is very much a mental one. If you have a strong mind, you can have a strong body image, you just need someone to empower you and this can start with parenting. My son did that for me. I knew I couldn't set a bad example for him and I am so very aware of the way I was brought up and how it affected me negatively so it made me determined for him not to go through the same experience. I also love reading books about real life experiences that inspire me to make the most of life and achieve things I never thought were possible. People like Sean Conway & Meredith Atwood really inspire me, real and ordinary people who have done extraordinary things.

Body Stories

Harpreet Chana
Mental Wealth Academy

I first became aware of my body image when I was six years old. We had just been on our first family holiday to India and I remember getting a real case of 'Delhi belly' whilst I was out there, alongside numerous members of my family. Everyone else had lost weight when they came back apart from me - I had been four stones something before I left and when I came back I was over five stones… At the age of almost seven.

I remember thinking, *Oh my god, I am so fat, what is wrong with me?* So, when everyone in my family was comparing how much weight they had lost in India, I didn't tell anyone that I had actually put on weight, as I was too ashamed. What I should probably tell you is that I was ridiculously tall for my age. I was easily a head above everyone else in my class. But the damage was already done. This is where I started to believe that I was fat and my negative body image began.

Fast forward a few years and I was now ten. I was being bullied by a group of girls in my class who were much smaller than me and made fun of my size. I distinctly remember a maths lesson where we were all being weighed at the front of the class and my teacher making everyone stop what they were doing as she exclaimed, 'Oh my goodness everyone, Harpreet weighs as much as 60 bags of sugar (60kg) and isn't that awful?' I was 5' 8" inches at the time and 60kg (9st 6lb) is a perfectly healthy weight for someone of that size.

But again, the damage was done and I spent the rest of my school days feeling fat, heavy, big and unattractive. What was worse, this and the bullying led me to start eating sugar in secret.

We didn't have much sugar in our house growing up. Sweets, chocolates and biscuits were a treat and following an awful visit to the dentist when I was quite young with my father (ironically the only visit he ever came to), my Dad effectively 'banned' me from sugar. As I now realise (and as a mother myself), the minute you forbid anything, that is exactly what the child will want more than anything else. And boy, did I! Every night after dinner I would sneak up to my room and eat sweets and chocolate which I would have bought with money from doing household work for a nearby relative.

Pretty soon, my weight started to increase. My mum couldn't figure out why this was happening as we generally ate a mundane diet of vegetable Curry and chapattis every day. Sugar became my emotional crux and all through school and exam life, I turned to sugar to provide me comfort. This resulted in me leaving school at 18 weighing nearly 13 stones.

This only got worse at University (as it does for most people who are living on a diet of cheap alcopops and late-night kebabs!) In 2004 I weighed more than ever and began yo-yo dieting in an attempt to lose weight and 'feel better about myself'. What I didn't realise, is that no matter how much weight I lost, I would put it back on again (and then some!), I never did feel better. In fact the whole diet-binge cycle just made me feel so much worse about myself because added to the emotion of feeling fat and unattractive, I now had feelings of disappointment that I couldn't do it and that I'd let myself down. Which would inevitably result in more eating, to provide comfort and more weight gain.

Then, two years ago, I started working with a mindset coach who for the first time, got me to appreciate and love my body, exactly how it is, by making me look at my naked body in the mirror and say what I loved about it. It was hard at first but so effective that I now get my clients to do the same! I currently weigh more than I have ever done in my life but I can honestly say I'm also the most comfortable in my skin than I have ever been in my whole life too. Because I am now no longer looking to lose weight to 'feel better about myself'. That is already there, within me.

In the last few months I have naturally started to lose weight from eating less, moving more and reducing sugar. Nothing more exciting than that. It truly is what works. But unless we can address the reason why we eat in the first place and start with a positive body image, we will always fail. I only wish I could go back and tell my six-year-old self that!

My Body, My Life, Continued…

Age 18

'Well… what did you get?'

'Not what I need. Sheffield have rejected me.'

Studying my A-levels had been the best time in my life so far. I jettisoned our local school as soon as I could and registered at the college in Solihull. It felt, to me at least, pretty bohemian. Ah, now I understood, *here* are my people. Whether it was the mixology of students or simply the age that we'd reached, education once again seemed like a safe place to be. How sad is that? I've never reflected on high school that way before.

But I'd enjoyed it too much. I'd had a job at a local Pizza Hut, Kitchen Supervisor, I had a car, an older boyfriend who I visited at Sheffield Uni, independence, big houses, often empty – so parties, and a good bunch of friends. But the 'B' I needed in French to study Oriental Languages at Sheffield let me down. It's not that I hadn't studied but my French was a shoe-in. I chose to revise my weaker subjects of Psychology and Philosophy - B and C respectively. A level results day was the day I got my first grey hair.

So come September, instead of studying languages I found myself through the clearing system, heading to Northumbria University to study Sociology and Criminology. There's a sizeable chance you wouldn't be reading this book if that hadn't happened.

Age 19

'KATIE!... I need help!'

My first term at Uni was pants, I was housed with the wrong people. But one day I met a camel-coat girl on a cold-breath morning, on a metro platform, Katie. She made life better then and has basically done that ever since. She has an easy way around life. She's witty and clever and isn't put off by weird, rabbit-hole questions or ideas. She taught me how to laugh at myself, to lighten up.

As luck would have it, one of her flat mates in halls didn't work out and I was able to take her room. Thank God! Uni got better after that. A group of six of us stayed together for the following two years in a house in Glenthorn Road, Jesmond. We drank and smoked a lot, watched daytime TV a lot, spent our grants like pocket money, had I *think* six hours of lectures a week. We had themed parties and food fights and trips to the beach. We pretty much rubbed along well together.

Then one day we were perusing the shelves of *Boots* and I said 'I'm going to try it!'

Getting it on was the easy part. When it came to ripping it off, it was like trying to swallow multiple times in a row. My body just wouldn't do it.

Katie burst into my room, 'What is it… *Oh*!'

'I tried but I just can't get it off!' I was lying prone on the bed, a wax strip flapping from my fou fou.

'OhmyGodithurtssomuch! How am I going to *get it off*? STOP laughing!'

There was some deliberation over angles and technique and many collapses into hysteria.

'Why would we do this to ourselves?'

'Just stay still!'

'You're just going to have to rip it…'

'Aaaaaaaaaaaaggggggh.'

Yikes! It was breath-taking and not in a good way.

'What are we going to do about the other side?'

Years later, after I was trained in epilation I would routinely wax my own vajayjay. There's nothing quite like your first time! Or a stuck-in-hot-water-situation to seal a friendship.

Age 20

'You're the Editor?'

'Err, yes', and other lessons in not having a clue what I'm doing!

My housemates and I had all been writers on *Newcastle Student*, the imaginatively-named student newspaper. I had taken on the role of Editor, the paper having no one else to do it and myself, no idea what an editor does. I just knew I loved to write. But I had what you would now call imposter syndrome. One thing I should have mentioned was I was a Sociology student living in a house full of English Literature undergrads. Who was I to run the paper? But I did have a lot of free time and I enjoyed going into the office and learning about it. I didn't however have the hubris, the easy manner or the skills to lead the others and felt totally out of my depth. I started having busy dreams and fitful nights. Instead of researching 'How to be an Editor', I went and sought counselling for my unsettling self-doubt and frankly it was overdue. It was the beginning of a long and rewarding relationship between me and talking therapies.

In writing this memory, I flicked back through my old cuttings and articles. In April 1999 I authored an article titled *Fat is Back* which I'd *completely* forgotten about:

'We all know that "super model" does quite literally mean superhuman, for what we see before us (in the media) is pure fantasy.'

'For women it (reality checking imagery) is a crucial mechanism of growing up.'

'The ultimate answer, is to market fat better.'

'What can we do? We can stop kidding ourselves. No more 'that woman is thin, and she uses that product, so if I use it…' and don't say you don't do it because if you didn't it wouldn't work as an advertising ploy and it obviously does.'

It is cringeworthingly crude but I am *so* happy to have found this article. Proof that this matter has been bothering me for over *twenty years!*

Age 21

In addition to my degree, my part time job at the cinema, my Editorship, I also volunteered at a writing charity in Newcastle and took part as a volunteer at the *Durham Literature Festival* before I left the North East. It was so eye-opening. I got to interview best-selling authors, helped run events for and had dinner with: Toby Litt, Darren Star, Amy Jenkins, Geoff Dyer, Jake Arnott, Will Self and Andrew Motion - Poet Laureate 1999-2009. It was fascinating learning about the publishing industry and feeling a part of that scene. It started my obsession with getting books signed. I totally winged it - I remember one time being asked what I'd like from the coffee shop and getting cappuccino mixed up with espresso.

'Really? You drink espresso?'

'Sure!' as I choked it down. What twenty-one-year-old drinks espresso?

At the end of my placement, I was given a thank you and goodbye from the team as they sent me off to London with a farewell comment: 'You know… you'll never be an author… you're too… normal.'

I was writing my first book so it came as a blow. Was I *too normal?* I drank espresso for God's sake! Also, they were right. Since then I have had many respected writers tell me that while I'm a good writer, I write safe characters. I *was* compliant, trained in seeking approval, I modelled normal. But…life had other plans for me…

I graduated with a respectable 2:1 but I knew I wanted to write so I left Newcastle and headed straight to London, where the streets are paved with vomit and needles. Or at least they were in the part I could afford to live. The flat was damp and cloying. I found a dead rat in my washing basket.

I started by doing work experience, first at *Company* magazine, then with *Sky*, not the media company, the then unisex style magazine. The *Sky* Editor, was pleased with my work, I got two weeks of work there to cover the Editorial Assistant's holiday. But then, nothing. I took on temp jobs that took me all over the city, to streets not lined with vomit and needles. Pimlico's nice! Mostly boring office work. I remember feeling pretty desperate. Then one day, I got a phone call. A magazine was looking for an Editorial Assistant. The Editor had put me forward. The pay was rubbish (for London) but I'd got my first real job. I was *so* excited!

I was sorting newspapers, delivering messages, sending packages, getting photos printed, but also writing film and TV reviews, clubbing at weekends, reviewing those, arranging vox pops, loads of freebies. The magazine was the biggest-selling young women's magazine in the UK. It was a fortnightly, pitched for 16-24-year-olds. It was most known for its 'Position of the Fortnight', a feature which schoolgirls would huddle round and giggle.

One of my jobs was to compile a fortnightly feature of topless men called 'Men Unzipped'. It was usually a sports team or club and it would involve me finding the men, taking a disposable camera and a notepad and asking them all the same question e.g.: 'Do you like long distance lovin' or a sprint finish?' Bleugh.

Looking back now, the content was so childish and objectifying. I did compile some features and put them forward but I'm not proud of them. They had bitchy undertones and had to have a sexual or just fake angle. There was no support or career progression. It is such a competitive industry that it didn't matter that this wasn't really for me, you have to start somewhere. I was mostly focussed on my own work and writing my own book, which I did before work, getting up at 6am.

One day I was in a team meeting room for some reason, probably bringing coffee. I was listening to the team talk about the demographic of the mag. Something like…

'But what are 16-to-24-year-olds *in to* right now?'

It wasn't my place but something pushed me to pipe up.

'But we know it's not though, right?'

The room looked at me. Senior Editors mostly. 'Sorry?'

'Well I mean' laughing 'we all know it's schoolgirls who buy it.'

I didn't say, *not one of my twenty-one-year-old friends read this or would have been seen dead with it.* We were all being paid with schoolgirl's pocket money!

'The magazine is pitched at this age range, if younger girls are getting hold of it, their parents really need to be taking responsibility.'

And that was that, the responsibility for the bodies and sex lives of under-age girls relinquished.

Still age 21

Did you know the pre-frontal cortex in the brain helps moderate social behaviour and emotional regulation? Interestingly it's also associated with interpreting reality – so there's a problem that fantasy bodies might pose there. The age of 25 is when most neurologists say the pre-frontal cortex is fully developed and as such is associated with reaching adulthood and maturity. Mine snapped into place at twenty-one. I remember it happening.

'You don't have to go in there to cry you know.'

I looked at myself in the mirror and paused squeezing the spot. I was in the bathroom of a Harley Street Hospital patient room. My Dad was the patient, he'd just had gall stones removed. I'd been in the room when the consultant gave the news. 'Routine lung scan, found a tumour'. But to me it was a bit like an MOT assessment, 'Yeah, definitely needs new wheels, so you're going to have to bring him back in'. I slowly went back into his room. 'Why… would I be crying?'

It must have been my pre-frontal cortex because my brain snapped Dad into the centre and shoved me out the side. I guess for the first time I wasn't the main focus of my life.

Days after that, became a routine of spending the day at work on the magazine, where I was on the radar of an irksome bully (wish I'd complained), followed at 6pm by me bussing the length of Oxford Street, up to Lancaster Gate. Dad was no longer a GP but a doctor working in the corporate world. In the 90s he was a front-runner in helping the corporate world get to grips with Occupational Health, would travel all over the world sharing his knowledge and vision and informing the government. At the time he was Global Medical Director at *Conoco* and they were putting Mum and Dad up in a swanky flat, while Dad received his treatment. At the end of the day I'd finally head home to my hovel to do it all again tomorrow.

Dad is one of the tiny population of men who get lung cancer but haven't smoked. I stopped immediately. He underwent surgery to remove two lobes of his lung. I saw him as he was wheeled out, still unconscious, surrounded by tubes. It was awful. My invincible Dad, my hero, reduced. The thought of losing him was the worst thing, my biggest fear. He was for me, my supporter, he got me, he talked to me about deep, rabbit-hole things. But he had chemo and he recovered. He took early retirement and returned to his life with Mum in Normandy, France.

Age 22

'I'm not asking you, I'm telling you, you *have* to leave that job. You are miserable!'

'Do you mean leave London?'

'You could do. You could come and live with us in France or you could go and stay with Aunty Aileen if you want to stay in England.'

It was such a hard choice. This was a 'dream job'. I got paid to go to the *Smash Hits Poll Winner's Party* and interview Kylie! (Actually I had to do that on a Sunday so maybe not strictly paid.) As an aside I had been asked by the team to ask her just one question: 'What's it like having the hottest bum in showbiz?' (This was the era of *Spinning Around* and the gold hotpants.) She faltered at the banal question and brushed it away. What I *do* remember though is the disposable camera I'd been given, wasn't working and she stopped what she was doing reached out and tried to help me fix it. She was genuinely lovely.

I was *so* disenchanted with work though. The unreality of it all. I wanted to produce gritty, intelligent content. And the way bodies were commodified was just so warped. The office did not reflect the magazine. The Fashion and Beauty Departments did more so. But the rest, Design, Features, Subs, Senior Management, all displayed the *real* diversity of bodies.

I also couldn't come up with any features ideas and I stopped trying. Maybe I should have swapped to newspapers, but that wasn't where I wanted to be either. I just couldn't unscrew my head enough to be able to create the content or the voice. I find a lot of media such a bag of skewed nonsense, I knew that wasn't what I wanted to be doing. I'd seen colleagues publish their own books and move on but I'd finished my book and made a new book out of the volume of publishing house rejections I'd got.

The bully I mentioned epitomised everything that was wrong with this media world. He performed the brand of snark that only men can publicly pull off, women would be crucified for it. Every day was an exercise in pretentious elitism and affected judgement, from food choices, to clothes, to his running commentary. It was toxic and exhausting and I imagine not all that unusual in fashion / media / creative offices. But still, I wasn't going to just throw in the towel. Then, one day I got a phone call.

Every magazine has a media pack. It's mostly for school kids looking to complete media projects, it would feature circulation, target audience figures, stuff like that. One of my jobs was to send that out to anyone who enquired about one.

'Oh hi, could you tell me who takes media enquiries please?'

'I can do that, what can I help you with?'

'Can you tell me your target demographic please?'

'Yes it's young women age 16 to 24 years-old. Shall I send you a media pack?'

'No that won't be necessary. Do you think that's accurate?'

'Oh, er… which bit?'

'The target audience. I mean, what about the magazine getting into younger hands?'

'Well it's really up to the parents to monitor that kind of thing…'

As I replaced the phone back in the cradle, I felt an unease rise like a tide. That wasn't a usual media request. Something was off. I took it to my Editor and admitted I thought I might have just accidentally given a quote for something.

Sure enough a scandal piece came out the following day in a tabloid newspaper, holding magazines like ours accountable (I haven't kept it!) with my words as 'a spokesman' and a cloud of shame gathered over my head. It followed me around the office. It probably could have dissipated but, I was done. Defeated.

The Editor wrote a complimentary memo to announce my departure. At my leaving drinks I thanked everyone and told them I would miss them. The man who had been feeding me snarky comments and bitchy bon mots for the duration of my time piped up and said 'How much love is there in this room?' It was a reference to Darius from Pop Idol and had been his comment following being dismissed from the show. It was a comment that had been hashed and rehashed by the press and Darius had been packaged as somewhat of a buffoon. So although it sounds innocent enough, kind even, and maybe it was just for a laugh, my final memory of the job was stained, embarrassed and eugh, that man! Later in life, perhaps I could have verbally sparred with this guy, and he would have respected it, we would have been friends. But because I was too young, or naïve or unLondon, all of his comments just landed badly. I should never have been there. I headed back to my family, back to Newcastle. In retrospect maybe my pre-frontal cortex wasn't quite all there!

Age 23

'It's come back pet.'

Aunty Aileen found me crying on the bedroom floor. Mum and Dad returned to the UK for his care. Back to a village I'd lived in between the ages of nine and 13.

'Will you come home?'

In the hospital I made a real hash of taking off his breathing mask, got it caught on his glasses. 'I'm not doing a very good job of being your nurse!'

'You're doing a great job pet.'

These are the last words I remember him saying to me. The essence of him to me. The one who was *for* me, encouraging me, who could tell me I'd done a good job… and I'd believe him.

He died on a hot day, in July 2003. Disobedient weather. And it felt so otherworldly, impossible, numb. It's hard to write through all these tears. I don't think about this much now, in honour of him. He'd hate me to be too sad, too much. Also as I'm writing Alexa stopped mid-song and started playing 'Fix you', which Chris Martin wrote for Gwyneth I believe on the death of her father. It's totally weird because Alexa is streaming my phone.

Things that helped were my bizarre, non-believing faith that I'll be with him one day and if not that we are attached through the rest of this life. That he is part of me. That I had an amazing Dad for 24 years.

Writing. I wrote loads trying to process it. I've never revisited the work. And in some kind of gift from the Universe, as he was leaving, another extraordinary man was entering my life.

Things that didn't help. Seeing him after, open mouthed, gone. I wish I hadn't, he wasn't there. Time didn't help. It went so slowly as I was healing, couldn't hurry up that process. It *was* the worst thing that could ever happen to me. If I could get through this then, there would be strength in that, I could get through anything. My body denied that Dad had gone and every morning it woke up optimistic, before the reality sank in. I remember wondering how many times this would have to happen before body would catch up with the new reality.

I'd been so distracted by Dad that I almost hadn't noticed I'd fallen in love. I imagine it's not easy trying to fall in love with somebody who's grieving. Nusband (not my husband) likes a challenge though, and I've been challenging him ever since. When you know, you know. We'd been dating just four months before we moved in together, two months more before we lost Dad… and ten months before we bought our first house together. He has an incredible amount of affection and love, empathy and concern – he takes care of business while always knowing the right thing to do and he was a big part of the recovery for me. Within two years together we'd bought our second house. We both had siblings who encouraged us to think about a family: 'It takes longer than you think, you might as well get on with it!'

But it didn't take long, in fact it happened immediately. It wasn't ideal. I had retrained at night school while I was temping in the day and I was building a business in holistic and beauty treatments. I worked out of one half of our new home, while we lived in the other. As the youngest of my siblings, I would be the first to start a family. I left the pregnancy test in the bathroom for him to find. He was so excited, we were both shocked but giddy. It felt too soon, I was like a rabbit caught in headlights…

Age 27 – Valentine's Day

'I'm sorry there's no heartbeat.'

I'd been so unsure and anxious about this pregnancy. I wasn't ready, but then I know everyone says… 'You're never ready.' The miscarriage was left to come away naturally, like a period. I was twelve weeks pregnant and it's true, once you've had a miscarriage, you realise so many others have had them too. Another body thing we never talk about! It's estimated that one in eight pregnancies end in miscarriage.

It wasn't that I was too sentimental about having lost my baby, it was more a general sense of loss. A plan that must be re-written, hope that has gone. I had been given a taste of pregnancy and I knew it wasn't really my cup of tea. Hormones raging, nausea and incredible tiredness. A helpful friend pointed out, 'Well you do literally have a parasite living in your body.'

Actually here's another thing we don't focus on when we're pregnant. Pregnant women are building humans. I don't know what I was expecting or how easy I thought that would be! Mum got a book for me: *Your Pregnancy Day by Day* by Stuart Campbell. It helped to remember the little accomplishments, ah today we're making fingernails…

But now, I was back to day zero. No fingernails made. Alright maybe I *was* a bit sentimental. Minus zero even, by who knows how long. Nusband and I licked our wounds and I comforted myself with the thought that at least the natural order could be restored, and my sister could lead the way with motherhood. That bit felt more right. We'll just try again. There were pregnant women *everywhere!*

My next period came and went, then the next, and the next. Each time I sunk lower and lower. Why is this not working? What was I getting wrong? Well *now* I wanted a baby! Suddenly I'd gone from being a bit blasé about wanting a baby to being acutely obsessed. I truly wanted this and was not only not been able to achieve it but felt a complete powerlessness over its outcome. I'd assumed this would be something I could control. Lack of control mixed with mounting panic, a sense of uselessness and low self-esteem left me slammed.

Sixteen months. Sixteen attempts. Sixteen defeats. Sixteen disappointments. Then one day I was chatting to one of my clients during her reflexology treatment. She was asking about children and I opened up to her about my struggle.

'Have you heard of the cervical mucus test?'

'No, what's that?'

Cervical mucus is the body's natural way of letting you know when it's ovulating. Basically (warning, this bit's a bit grim) the discharge that a woman makes in her vagina, becomes a bit like slime for a few days of the month. It should be stretchy and if handled will stretch from your thumb to your middle finger without breaking, at our most fertile time. Nature's lube! Go body! Ergo, it indicates when you should be having sex in order to get pregnant. Disclaimer: **You can also get pregnant at other times, it's just a natural signal.**

'So look out for that', my client advised. So I did.

I realised that the emotional roller coaster I'd been on had a pattern. The days leading up to a period would bubble with excitement. Then bleeding. Then sunken disappointment. Then rampant love-making. This would last all of about a week because honestly who can keep it up. Fatigue would set in, so we'd conclude we'd done enough and take a break (clearly I could have listened more in biology class!). If this cervical mucus thing was right, we'd have been on the hiatus period of the routine, right when really we should have been bonking all night long! We tried this new approach and the following month, after all those missed months, we scored! And that proud, nauseous, dog-tired, head mash of a pregnancy, was mine!

What I'd like us to take from this is (a) how clever are our bodies? It had been trying to tell me all along. And (b) why the hell don't we talk about these things? While I agonised about it with family and friends for almost a year and half, could no one tell me there's this really clever signal and it works! I think it's because we don't talk about bodies that way, because we don't worship them and value them for the flipping mega star, super-heroes they are! Because we're squeamish or prudish or because simply, we don't know. I have read a lot of women's magazines and never read *anything* about it. Because the value in our bodies has never been around what incredible pieces of kit they are. Who would profit from that? What would be the point of that?

Only in planting an insecurity attached to a problem-solving product do our bodies perform any social value… apparently.

Age 28

'Yeah I know but I really think we need to go.'

'We don't. I've just got into bed!'

'Yes but I read here that something called *ruptured waters* can happen and when I've just stood up from the bath, it feels like it's… coming out of me.'

'Babe you're 24 weeks, it's fine. You're not going to read about *ruptured waters* and then hey presto you've got ruptured waters. Also water is running off you from the bath. Come to bed, I've been at work all day!'

It was also his birthday…

'We'll be driving *back* along this road in half an hour', he grumbled as he rubbed his forehead and sighed.

In half an hour we were blue-lighted to another hospital, where they had incubators to take babies as small as ours if this was him deciding to make an entrance because guess what? My waters had ruptured. At this stage, it was safer to try and keep him in as long as possible. There was a risk of infection as his safe-haven had been breached but getting him out at this early stage was riskier still. The following morning, early, before Nusband had arrived back at the hospital, a doctor came to see me with a form.

'Is it OK if I ask you some questions?'

'Yes, no problem.' I wasn't prepared.

'…If this baby *does* want to make an entrance early… do you want us to go to *all lengths possible* to save him?'

'Well yes, of course!' Nusband should have been here for this. Why didn't they wait?

'Now I urge you to take a little while to think about this.'

'There's nothing to think about.'

'...It could mean you living with a child with a severely limited life. It could mean they would never be able to walk, talk, they could be incontinent into adulthood or they could die young. I'm sorry that this is a difficult conversation, but it is part of my job to make you aware of all the eventualities.'

I took a deep breath. I still didn't truly understand the enormity of what was being asked. And they wanted an answer, now... on my own.

I replied, 'Yes, please save him.'

I spent a week over Christmas in hospital, quietly committing to doing something for parents whose kids are sick, because this was *awful* and I hadn't even met him yet! My mother-in-law sent in a Christmas dinner. I closed my business, lay down for the remaining 16 weeks and my body - because it's a flipping clever piece of kit - healed itself and replenished the amniotic fluid while it was at it. You know where this is going... flipping incredible my body!

Years later, doing voluntary work at a children's hospice, I'd have the opportunity to reflect more on the enormity of that decision. How the care for a child with extreme life limitations not only eclipses one's own life, needs, relationships but can be a challenge to your very soul. It can be a life of little griefs and mutual suffering that might add up to much more than the initial grief of losing a newborn. But in that moment, there's nothing the doctor could have said to make me understand. I write this only to offer my honest opinion. As with many controversial things, this is a simplistic and generalised view. There are some incredible parents out there with the ready skills and tender care to cope and thrive under these conditions. I do mean extreme life limitations where basic self-care or personal expression are prohibited. However there are also parents out there who carry the weight of guilt at not being able to save a baby, or who let nature take its course rather than step in, or who perhaps will perceive a termination as a failing, rather than a kindness. Society is not giving them permission to be at peace with the decision. I've seen the care of a child with severe life limitations break families, break people. We live in a culture that saves lives at all cost. I know I blamed myself for the miscarriages, blamed my body for not being able to hold on to my babies. In hindsight, maybe my body gave me a kindness too. This is hard to write, I'm not an expert, only an observer, but if it gives a family (or a lone woman in a hospital bed) pause before making such an immense and pressurised decision, then it's worth it. On further reflection before my work at the hospice and candid conversations with parents, all of my knowledge on this came from the media. Dramatised versions of events where people overcome abject adversity and thrive. My saying 'save him' was based on many versions of the story where it is the 'right thing to do'. I think the doctor that day was gently trying to infer the enormity of the decision, still I guess nothing she could have said would have changed my answer.

Age 29

'I'm going to poo, I'M GOING TO POO!'

The ruptured waters had been closely monitored but stable for fifteen and half weeks. Then one day, sat in a carpet showroom car park, I felt that familiar trickle again.

They induced me at 39 weeks and four days. Another overnight stay. I'd just switched off the TV in an attempt to settle down for the night when I heard a pop! Felt a gush.

The body doesn't remember pain (because it's genius – and thank God!) so there's not a lot I can tell you here apart from, yes it's called labour for a reason, yes I wanted it to be over, I panicked, asked for more drugs than I was allowed, my body started involuntarily shaking when I transitioned to the final stage of labour. I know that birthing a human feels like you need an enormous dump which on reflection… of course it does! I know it *is* possible even when it feels like something must be very wrong or that it simply won't work. I remember only needing to do four pushes and it was over, that the really tough bit was only right at the end but not having done this before, I didn't realise that at the time.

They don't tell you any of that on adverts for milk or nappies! In fact culturally, because we don't talk about these things, childbirth is packaged as blissful, glowing, heart-warming, instant maternal connection and instinct. Society doesn't package it as trauma. I asked Aunty Aileen afterwards, 'Why does nobody tell you?'

'Because you'd never do it if we did.'

She might have a point there and what an enormous loss that would be. I wonder how many days of pain I would endure to have my kids? Probably quite a few. Luckily I only had to do it for one day of my life for each of them. That's a pretty good return I think. I've endured longer pain for my dog but that's another story! Also, it's an absolute travesty that women are in any way side-lined in this world. But institutionalised sexism aside, women are flipping warriors! Miracle workers of the highest order. They should be *worshipped* and I think maybe that's what scares the boys.

So I'm lying there in hospital, my baby still lying foetal on me, his feet making tiny red footprints on my chest feeling both numb and absolutely overwhelmed. I didn't feel an instant connection - I'd only just met this dude! I vividly remember thinking, *one day, he'll have a beard and he'll need to learn how to drive, and I need to get him from here to there!*

But within days that changed. I mooned over him sleeping for hours. I loved him with so much of myself that somehow it hurt. How could love *hurt* like that? Months into our relationship I remember thinking, *it's like someone has given me the crown jewels and I have to keep them safe, but not in a bank safe or a vault, out in the world.* I *have to take the crown jewels with me everywhere I go, or worse! Trust someone else to not lose them or break them!* Relaxing much!

Looking back through a twelve-year window it's easy to see what was happening. Losing my Dad in fact hadn't been the hardest thing that would ever happen to me. Losing my child would be. And I'd already carelessly lost one! Around this time, I also knew two families who had tragically lost their full-term babies, to Sudden Infant Death Syndrome. On top of the miscarriage, the ruptured waters and Dad it felt like my baby's life was so fragile, I felt so anxious of anything taking him away from me.

However at the time, I couldn't see anything abnormal about it. And anyway I was busy learning to Mum while keeping an eye on something else, his sibling. I never wanted a big gap between my kids and I didn't want him to be our only child, so I attended to the business in hand of building us another human so that I could close the door on this baby-making chapter.

So good was our understanding of the cervical mucus test, we had our next 'bundle of joy' on the way by August of the same year. I don't 'put that in quotes' to imply he wasn't pure joy. He was so gorgeous, it's just what I was feeling wasn't joy… and that sort of narrative must have been written by a man… or more likely a nan, far far away from the reality.

However once again the Universe knew better than us, perhaps saved us from a larger grief and we lost that baby too in the November. I was left to miscarry myself again and this time it wasn't slow like a period but laboured into the toilet while a family dinner went cold. Another sadness, increased anxiety, but there was no lengthy wait and in January 2010 in a labour that was much less fearful and as such felt more in my control, The Girl One arrived to complete our family. Another set of crown jewels.

It gave me the opportunity to reflect. On this second birth I went somewhere else with my deep breathing, that just made the whole thing flow better. I didn't panic so much because I knew what to expect and I felt otherworldly and a little bit absent using just my breath and some gas and air. I trusted my body to do the work. It was a waterbirth and in total irony, this one came out *in* her bag. The midwife had to pop it! My daughter was lifted into my arms and I sank back against the plastic bath and closed my eyes, not in maternal euphoria as it might have been assumed but in gratitude to the Universe that the hardest physical thing I'd have to do in my life was behind me. Also... I really should be careful what I thank the Universe for!

Some time passed and I realised something. Every time the kids did something super-cute or memory worthy, my mind would instantly jump to the thought, *please don't die.* To begin with that was just a feeling and I hadn't been able to put it into words. Then as time went on, it's like it was actually a little voice in my head. Which made it easier to engage with. I remember being at the top of our stairs with those two little monkeys, messing about doing something, being the cutest and this voice pipes up. It was the last time I let it. I sat down and thought to myself, I *have* to move this thought out of my head. These babies were rough, tough, robust little bundles of joy. I wondered how I would do that and I thought back to my Dad. The time had tempered my grief and I was now able to feel glad that I'd had him in my life, some people don't even *have a dad.* Maybe I could do the same here. So going forward every time I felt that feeling of pride and uber-cuteness I was glad to have had the experience of it. To have had these babies for as long as I had. To be sharing my life with them. It was the beginning of a relationship with gratitude that is a very strong part of me now.

Gratitude helps us to face an uncertain future. It helps us to notice the little wins and joys in life. If we know we're going to have to write down our gratitudes, perhaps at the end of the day, it makes us search our lives for them, rather than just endure what happens to us. It can change a pessimist into an optimist, and it forms the basis of satisfaction training (more on that later). Literally two minutes a day can do all that.

I had been so anxious. I hadn't realised and probably wouldn't have admitted it, such is the stigma. I had a wonderful health visitor. But because it wasn't outwardly interfering with my life, and it was so important to me to be succeeding at mothering, it went under the radar for us all. But gratitude, along with some other skills I picked up on the way, has paved a path to happiness and it shores me up when the storm comes in. It is the best piece of advice I have. Get grateful, make it a habit, craft it into a talent and before long it will be who you are and pay you back in ways you can't imagine. I get to *enjoy* my tremendous kids, guilt and fear-free because of gratitude.

Age 33

'I know we said it was unlikely at your age; we were wrong. We *have* found a tumour.'

I remember taking it all on. Baby Girl at two-years-old was on my knee. I didn't cry, flinch, panic. I just listened. Then rang Nusband. I had been playing the game of, *if I ignore it, it will behave and go away*, so he'd forgotten where I was.

'I'm at the hospital, it's not what we'd hoped.'

'What's not?'

'It *is* cancer.'

I was sent for more biopsies, tiny painful pockets of my breast removed and analysed. The mastectomy was booked in. It was all happening so fast. I felt euphoric, my Breast Care Nurse assured me that was normal. I just thought I was coping really well! I now realise my body had shut its feelings, physical and emotional, down in order for me to cope. (It would be two more years before it would start to open again in a grief-stricken, angry whorl. Look after your cancer survivors years later please.)

I remember thinking, *Kylie's fine. Be like Kylie.* I remember thinking *Thank God I'll get a rest.* Which gives you an idea of the state of my life at that time. Trying to achieve everything, make my mark, raise two kids, be great at it while creating a booming business. There was no space, no gaps, no breather, no me. This would give me, me back. And in a perverse way, I was *glad*!

From diaries:

One Lump or Two?

Five actually; cancerous tumours in my right boob. I tried a number of times yesterday to tell The Boy, four years old, something... anything. I don't even know what, but every time, the words morphed in my throat into something else.

My other concern is my boobs. A boob job has never been on my 'to do' list or even 'if I had the money' list. I have to make the decision between going flat and having the frame of a young boy (on reflection that would have been immensely less hassle) or a WAG. Then there's the chicken fillet option - I struggle with the faff of my contact lenses so I can't see that going down well. Another option was to use my back muscle to create a more natural pair of puppies, but operations back and front with further scarring and hello? Don't I need my back muscle? You see, not good options.

And then there's my hair, I have no problem shaving it off once chemo begins. I've had a skinhead / number 2 before in my college days, it's no biggy. But I don't know how to explain it to the kids - especially The Boy. He's pretty unforgiving of people's idiosyncrasies. At the baths the other day while waiting for the slide, he reached out to poke a fat man's overhang before I *thankfully* caught his hand!

Baby Girl is already sensing something. Since the hospital she has been closer than usual, saying 'Mummy, I'll keep after you', before promptly forgetting and setting off to admonish her brother about something. Actually... having cancer feels like nothing, I feel the same today as I did last week, last year, all my life. The irony being that when this killer is cut out and obliterated with drugs, I'll feel pretty shocking.

My BooBs are Killing Me!

My career has been as a body worker and I have training in energy work. I think because of that, my fight, if you want to call it that, is not with the cancer per say but with fear. In fact, it's not a battle with cancer, it's a no-nonsense, zero tolerance policy. You're fired my friend, now hop it. I'll kick you into next week. If you're looking for trouble, you've found it! And staying calm, unafraid, is my most vital healing weapon. I'm a big believer in feeling good to feel better. Note I say 'believer' - because staying calm isn't always me. I think this has shocked the hysteria out of me. Even I'm surprised how calm I feel! For information, my consultant later tells me she prefers to think of it, frame it as a journey not a fight or battle. That way… there are no losers, and she's right.

So I'm cheering myself on. I've commandeered an anthem: *Titanium,* by David Guetta ft Sia and I am speaking to my cancer frequently, letting it know in no uncertain terms, its days are numbered. I'm visualising tiny Vulcan Bombers flying over my chest, dropping bombs on enemy invaders. Or geysers behind them, against my chest wall, exploding out of my body taking all of the dirty matter with them. I used to think this body wasn't good enough. It wasn't... but not for the reasons I thought...

The kids are helping, they have no response to cancer. It's everyone else's responses that are freaking me out: fear, shock, sadness, outpourings of love, anger but my favourite is easily humour! I was unprepared for everyone wanting to see me, it soon became impractical. I prefer to be alone, to concentrate on visualisations and not being scared. There's a jam jar in my stomach, sometimes it opens and lets out a little panic, makes me feel sick, so I screw it tight shut again. I have wrangled over whether I should be freaking out and having more emotion about this or if I should stay calm. My choice is to stay calm for as long as I can. Will it hit me? It sort of does. *Titanium* comes on the radio one morning after I've dropped the kids off at school and nursery and I cry hard and quick at the chopping board in the kitchen... then I get on with the washing up.

When I have my surgery I will have a Sentinal Node Biopsy. This means some of my lymph nodes will be removed from my armpit to see if the cancer has spread beyond my breast. I visualise Pac Men eating away at my malignant cells. Barking, snarling, nasty dogs defending my lymph nodes. Virtual cling film around my boob preventing anything leaving it. Vacuum hoses at my lymph nodes, sucking anything back that might have got out.

I eventually tell The Boy. The conversation starts, as is so common these days, with us barking at each other, then... 'I need to tell you something Little Man. Mummy has a… bug in her boob', he summed it up perfectly:

'So this is a Super Boob, and soon this one will be too!'

'…That's right.' Years later he would sit through an assembly and really learn what it means to have cancer and that night his grief would flow.

I met an older lady at the hospital, we're going under the knife on the same day. She was there alone. I don't feel lonely. Nusband, my gorgeous Nusband, is proving himself, not that there was any doubt, to be my tower of strength. He improves the way I think... is making a positive person out of me. Two weeks following my diagnosis, I will have surgery to remove my right breast. I suddenly feel protective towards my boobs; my nipple. I like it, it's mine, but it has to go. It looks like a nipple and matches the other one! In fact I now realise I like my boobs in general (although in recent years they have taken on the role of droopy spaniels' ears adorned with stretch marks). They're familiar to me, I'll miss them. I immortalised them in plaster, it was an appropriate farewell. (I will later reflect that they are comfy in bed, I can lie on them, they support me).

And actually, the kids are at the perfect age for me to have cancer (weird sentence I never thought I'd write!) They're not old enough to understand but old enough not to wake us in the night or need their bums changing. Pretty self-sufficient all told, so best it's happening now. They also have no respect whatsoever for cancer which is hugely refreshing when that's all I have been talking about. They are an elixir, a world of utter distraction. And when I'm feeling tired and Baby Girl insists 'Mummy, sit up, stand up, now let's go shopping' which involves pretending to buy carrots in the dining room, I find myself doing it. And, of course, them, I can't leave them. I've got too much I need to teach them and learn from them and experience with them.

Then there's the other side of it. We spend the weekend after the diagnoses with some lovely friends. We have fun and try to forget the elephant in the room. Kathryn takes some beautiful pictures of the family, paparazzi style. They make me smile. I posted the pictures on the private Facebook page I've set up, to show everyone I was OK but later I imagine them in a montage at my funeral. I start to wonder what songs I'd like. Could it be *that* is the story? At the start of this journey, I don't know how it will end. I know there's no strength in these thoughts. Perhaps it will focus me more on living a better life, I can now see that life has been... pretty mediocre. In actual fact we have had a stressful ten years, starting with my Dad's death, two house moves, four pregnancies, two miscarriages and two business closures. Which to this I can now add personal injury / illness and it covers seven of the ten most stressful things to happen to a person. All I need now is a marriage, a divorce and a jail term and I'd have the full hit! But to get to enjoy my life, perhaps it is just the warning I needed. Hard times now, followed by a long and happy life. Yes please, can I choose that one?

Inflate-a-girl

So surgery... During assessment: 'You've put on weight since pre-assessment'.

'I've just got more clothes on' - defensive much? This from a man who was clearly, at this early hour, a smoker and my mind boggles at it. He deals with people potentially dying *every day* but is actively ruining his health. I felt angry even though I shouldn't.

Then into another room to meet with my consultant. I will be having a full mastectomy on my right side, replaced by an inflatable implant to stretch the skin. Then a port leading to just under the surface of the skin, where it can be filled up later (clever). And then an augment (small implant) on my left side to even things up. My consultant used surgical marker pen, to make a visual plan of the operation. I look odd afterwards, like someone's defaced me while I'm drunk, or one of the kids has got felt-tip happy while I've been catnapping. My stomach was liquid, I expressed some concern about this to my consultant, much like during child birth I was anxious about making a mess with my bodily fluids but she gently reassured me it was just nerves and that nothing like that would happen. My consultant is *so* lovely and that makes this hard thing easier. Then into another room to meet with the anaesthetist. I wished she'd smiled more. Her questions reminded me that I still have a twenty-year-old brace fitted on the back of my teeth... she made note, for the airway.

Mine was the first surgery of the day which I was thankful for but I still had to wait in ANOTHER room with two women having knee operations. A nurse came and put some surgical stockings on me and gave me a pillow. It was all getting a bit real now. The telly was on. Lorraine Kelly was all about *Breast Cancer Awareness*, I now know it's *Breast Cancer Awareness Month*! I was momentarily distracted as Gary Barlow was coming on but then they came to take me through to theatre before I could see it – rats!

The next room was an anteroom, it was all a bit too *Gray's Anatomy* - full of medical stuff. I reminded myself to take long, slow breaths. It was a small room only just fitting in a gurney which I climbed on to, consultant, nurses and an anaesthetist, with no room to spare. A cannula was inserted into the back of my hand, it took a couple of times for them to get it in. I was then rolled onto my side. I knew this was because they were going to put me under using the cannula and then inject my back with a block so I wouldn't feel anything. The anaesthetist keeps sniffing aggressively. That's the last thing I remember.

Then someone called my name. And it was done. Writing this, I'm welling up... and I just chatted with the nurse, who I later didn't recognise but she said we'd talked about ice skating! I had a look under the hospital gown, all I could see was bandages, it wasn't too freaky. One very nice left boob and some dressings where the other one had been. It didn't and still doesn't feel like there's anything missing. I noted with some relief, the presence of my own knickers, fully clean and intact!

I was taken up to the ward, Nusband arrived and I tried to sit up using my hands to push me but the pain party in my armpits soon made me realise that wouldn't be possible. I also had a pain in my right side - not where the boob was, it was down on my ribs. This is where there was a drain to remove liquid that might form around the site. There is also the port which will be used to inflate the currently flat implant. My consultant came to see me. She tells me that the pain in my side is because my muscles have been separated from my ribs; that'll do it I suppose. The drain was uncomfortable coming out, yowzers! The port in my side is the worst part of it as I'm slim and it rests on my ribs, under the skin. My consultant tells me that the cancer had come out contained and was not attached to the chest wall, which is great - my visualisations had clearly worked! But we still need to get the results of the sentinel node biopsy to see if it has spread.

Recovery

Sometimes it felt like the engorgement which happened when my milk came in after having the kids, sometimes pain nerves fire off momentarily and it hurts and as soon as it's come, it's gone. Mostly it just feels numb. I took myself off meds four days after the op.

From diaries : Had my bandages off today and actually not too shabby! In Nusband's words 'Not as much of a car crash as I was expecting' (I know he means it with love). The nurse taking off my dressings gasped 'You have beautifully healing skin!' Is she flirting with me? I had never considered super-healing skin as part of my skillset and yet here we are. My surgeon has done a beautiful job. So now I can have a bath, hurray! Later, when I'm alone, I undress. There is still the yellow pigment of ammonia covering the area and those pen marks. I look up into the mirror and see myself for the first time. It's a strange sensation, of course it is me, but I don't recognise myself. It looks like pain, but doesn't feel like it. And going forward, this is me now, or a version of me, there's no going back. So the question is Em, can you accept it? Can you be happy with this? It was a definite decision *and…* it was a yes – had to be really. What would be the point of fighting it? I was going to nurture this body and I made up my mind to only see strength. To feel proud.

Then within days I start to be able to sleep on my preferred right side as the port hurts less, the bruising goes down, the dressings come off, I can go to the toilet on my own! Get dressed on my own! Put my hair up, even reach the washing up liquid. I was pleased to get home, to my beautiful family. Nusband always teasing me and making me smile. God I love him so much. The Boy asks 'Are the boob bugs gone?', The Girl says, 'I love you more than butterflies'.

I keep toppling over in bed! You'd be surprised how much you rely on your boobs for balance! I am suffering from short-term memory loss, I've just forgotten the next thing! I do that a lot!

The good news is... there is no cancer in my lymph nodes which means it hasn't travelled. This news is huge! But... it could still be in my body so Project Chemo starts on Tuesday. Today has been about some complicated decisions. Temporary menopause now or chances of final early menopause caused by chemo. Opted for temporary menopause now - implant required tomorrow. Bad drugs or truly awful drugs to treat something that may or may not be there. I opted for the worst to start with but my Oncologist talked me out of it (you don't want to know). Chemo at two, or three week intervals, I've opted for two, no respite. Followed by 18 doses of Herceptin. This programme will take eighteen months.

It doesn't feel like boob has gone. There is a stump where it was but I'm not aware of it having gone when I'm not looking or touching it. I hadn't realised I was afraid of touching it until I did. It felt hard, very hard and alien to me. It's taking getting used to but besides a bit of bruising it's not too shabby!

I wish my phone would stop turning 'boob' into 'anna' in predictive text... Every time I take my clothes off, my boob has moved! Very disconcerting! But nice, like growing a sunflower, and worth the feeling of having a space hopper wedged where it shouldn't be! As it is an expander the idea is that it will shift and move down and also expand over time to be made bigger – to match the other one. I do feel tired and I can't do as much as I'd like but pain levels have generally been low. The nerves to my boobs were cut in the operation so just a numbness really. There are dimples in my boob as it changes, with a hard ridge at the bottom. Ahhh! I've just seen my pec muscle tense *over* my boob!

Front page news – 'There's a huge rise in breast cancer in young women'. Here's my theory: Stress – I know, ground-breaking. But brought on by modern living. We're the first generation to be fed so unremittingly this crapsticks about having to be *everything* while having 'The Lifestyle' to accompany it. We have to have a super job and be an awesome good Mum and have meaningful friendships, a deeply satisfying love life. The house, the car, the holidays, all perfect and in place. Anything else results in that question... where am I going wrong? Add to that - the inability to switch off from technology and a sense of just perpetual urgency. STRESS!!! The thing that can't easily be measured but would explain why some smokers live till they're a hundred and other non-smokers die when they're 57. The specialists say it's caused by binge drinking... perhaps... I don't drink often now, but I have been to uni. I am a normal specimen of my generation in that respect but there are worse drinkers out there than me roaming around cancer free. And on reflection, when I see a life that *is* too outwardly perfect, it rings alarm bells in me. Surely it can't be super healthy to be living up to such high standards all round, it may speak more of feelings of inadequacy and yet we totally glorify this state.

Inflation Day! So this is where a needle is inserted into the port on my ribcage and saline solution is injected into the, currently deflated, implant. The reason for this is to stretch the skin, because they've taken all mine and are probably using it as a cute snap purse on their days off. It will be *uncomfortable* for a couple of days

apparently.
Well let me tell you, I do NOT enjoy this sensation. I've never been shot, but I imagine this is how it might feel. Not pain wise, it doesn't hurt exactly, it just... feels like a ball has suddenly materialised inside your chest – which I appreciate is exactly what has happened. It feels like pressure, discomfort, like a squash ball is sort of snuggling down for hibernation among the warm folds of my anatomy and physiology. Still my body adapts, accepts, welcomes this new guest.

I'm missing loads of stuff. The Boy has *just* started school and there are all these things I can't do because of risk of infection: assemblies; a special lunch date the parents were invited to; parents evening. Moo! But then, Baby Girl: 'Mummy's my best friend' and The Boy miming 'I heart you'

Jaine Broscoe Price's Photography Studio

I had no idea why, but following my diagnosis, my instinct was to get naked in front of a camera!

Dear Jaine

This is going to be a strange email a bit out of the blue. We met last year, almost to the day, I gave you a reflexology treatment.
You told me you are a photographer specialising in women and babies and I am writing, wondering if you would like to be involved in a charity project I'm working on.
I have been diagnosed with breast cancer two weeks ago, I had my mastectomy on Tuesday and I am wondering if you would like to chart the changes that my body will go through over the coming months. I have a deflated implant where my boob used to be and it will be inflated over time, along with losing my hair and various

other changes. I thought periodical photos would be interesting and we might be able to sell the story and pics to a glossy mag for next years' *Breast Cancer Awareness Month* - which I now know is October! The money we raise from this could go back into Breast Cancer Charities.

I am having my first inflation on Wednesday, which I know is a bit soon, the idea only occurred to me today.

Anyway, if you do feel like it might be something you'd be interested in / have any ideas for, please don't hesitate to contact me.

Best wishes

Emi

Two days later I got a reply…

Hi Emi

I am so sorry to hear of the recent, dramatic changes to your life.

Yes, of course I will work with you on this – no question about it.

I shall call you later to see what we can arrange pre-Wednesday ... and will discuss how we can use this situation to help others, and yourself.

You have my total support.

Speak later

Jaine

And so we began. Jaine always asked me for my creative input prior to shooting. On the first shoot I had this idea of taking chewing gum and looking all like 'What?' and nonchalant in the pictures, with my severed boob. It didn't work. In the finished image I look sad and distracted and not the least bit nonchalant. We picked a word to sum up my feelings for every shoot too. For this first one I chose 'Uneasy', because I had no real idea how the next few months / years of my life were going to work out. I felt uneasy about what would unfold, but I also suspected it would also *not* be easy.

At this point the reason for doing the project was because there should be a place where newly diagnosed folks can see what's ahead, ready themselves for the changes that are going to occur to their bodies. There are two modes of thinking here, I know. Some folks may want to bury their head or not want fearful images in their minds. But it was what I wanted. I wanted to see that it would all work out ok. Thankfully it did. You can now see the finished project on Instagram @thecancernude.

That's why I thought I did it anyway. In fact the real reason didn't present itself for many years...

I love the smell of chemo in the morning...

Before I started chemo I had some pretty wild preconceptions. I just thought it would be a growing constant pain, by the time I'd be finished I'd be the shell of a woman. I'd be grey, lifeless, in agony. It wasn't like that...

From diaries:

'I'm a bit worried about the side effects.'

My nurse: '...'

The chemo ward waiting area has a unique smell. I knew from having the kids that I hate cannulas. But also that it's just pain. Short-lived. So I get hooked up and off we go. As I'm sitting there, I'm trying really hard not to feel scared. To control my body, not succumb to rising anxiety. It feels like a tug of war. Physically it doesn't feel like much. An hour or so later, it's done. I can go and wait for whatever is going to happen… to happen.

At home, I'm lying down, hoping the chemo won't notice me. As time goes on, I feel tired and woozy with a headache, some mild nausea, offensive wind and a feeling of not quite being all there. It's a hangover. That's how it felt, like a hangover. No other side-effects, no mouth ulcers or constipation that I knew could happen, so I continue doing what I am doing and just see what happens. It's really odd, waiting for your body to react to something like this. I've become hyper-sensitive to myself! Is that…? Did that feel like…? I'm just trying to let it wash over me.

I decided to shave my hair off, I couldn't face it falling out and want to be in control of the experience. It's funny how one's goals change. I am *now* hoping my stubble won't fall out (because with it I looked like Ripley in Alien 3 and without it I'll look really ill) before our Annual Pie Off get-together this Friday. And to think once, perfecting my vintage roll was my biggest concern!

We shaved it off as a family, got my hairdresser to come to the house. Baby girl stood on my knee watching intently and we all laughed and made a joke of it. For the kids a funny, weird thing to do. Then later, The Boy One, who had just started school said… 'Mummy, I know it was funny, you shaving your hair off but… you're not going to go *to school* like that are you?' It was the first time I'd known him to be self-conscious or even self-aware. 'No darling, Mummy's going to wear a hat' … me choking back tears.

I guess no single thing is too bad and nothing seems to last for too long. The trick for me with the hard bits is to not deal with the big picture. Tiny steps, teeny ones, moments if necessary. 'Breathe. I can get through the next breath. Breathe. That was fine. Breathe. Made it through that one.' It's not all like this but there are times like this.

I go to the chemo support group, where I'm reminded I could die from chemo, that I will put on weight from the steroids, that I will be having more chemo than I thought and this won't be over by Christmas. My heart sinks. Not sure I can go to the group again. I feel like I can't support others. There's no room for me to support anyone else right now. I don't want a cancer friend… if I'm honest a cancer friend who might die. I couldn't cope!

November 2012

My farts should come with a toxic label! They absolutely stink! I wonder if that is what that weird smell was that first day in chemo? I hate that I look sick. I'm not sick. I've not got cancer. What you can see is the solution, not the problem but it looks undeniably cancerish! Make-up makes my eyes run like rivers.

Day one: OK until bedtime then nausea and a headache.

Day Two: OK until tea-time then a tiredness that rids me of my will to live. A little nausea and headache. No actual vomiting though (ever).

Day Three: A shocker – I've cried both Thursday mornings so far. Mum is here to support me with the kids, she's really stepped up. I keep telling her 'It's not as bad as it looks.' It doesn't hurt, I'm not being sick. I just can't function. Can't think, can't reason. My bones ache. But it's nothing worse than a major hangover and at its worst it's not longer than 24 hours. All of this 'poison' or 'attacking every cell' in my body... it's such dramatic imagery and language isn't it – it feels like a hangover to me. I was expecting worse. I can't drink enough, *so* thirsty, never feel satisfied but I can't drink too much at once either. I get pangs when I see women with long hair. It's going to take *years*!

The pubes are the first to go!

I'm losing my sense of humour, I've got to get it back. OK So it's not just that it feels like a hangover – it's that I'm losing my body. Seeing people is hard; not fun. It's depressing, I seem to have nothing else to talk about. Where has my life gone? Maybe I won't see people? I feel nauseous when I move, smell washing powder, smell my own body – my gases! And headaches... And I just feel myself is not here. It looks bad, laboured breathing, can't keep my eyes open. Sallow skin, hunched shoulders, no hair… My hair started coming out today in the shower – just the stubble that's left. Tiny hairs covering my breasts. Itchy. Nothing works in the hat department. Too hot, too cold, too itchy, and all of it looks too ill!

I read about a cancer survivor saying – there's nothing you can do, you have to leave it to the doctors and chemicals. I think that's rubbish, you can do a lot to help yourself. You can look after yourself, eat well, be sensible, you can think positive, work on you, be prepared to change.

I'm still baffled by the uncertainty of what my body will do next, but still no constipation or mouth ulcers etc. I like to think I'm helping myself. But when people use the word 'fatigue', it makes it sound like tiredness. It isn't tiredness, because sleep doesn't help it, a shower doesn't wake you up. A walk doesn't energise you. What I would give to feel refreshed. Feel alive! Water tastes like milk, milk tastes like water. Peanuts don't register at all. This taste change thing is the cruellest blow.

One of the markers I use to assess my state of mind and body, is whether I can gather myself enough to go and pop my head round the kid's bedroom door before I go to bed, give them a nuzzle. On this cycle, it took me six days to be back to mummying... I can't miss witnessing who they turn out to be. The thought of having to leave them makes me emotionally baulk. I realise what Dad had to go through to say goodbye.

I love living in the moment, sometimes that's all I can do. But with one good week and a bad one to follow, it's a good training camp for enjoying what you can. Also the contrast is great. Feeling good is so, *so* good compared to feeling chemo-tastic. Although good still isn't normal.

I'm on a new type of chemo and I almost broke the rule: there's no crying in chemo ward! That's not an actual rule, it's just a place of stoic, stiff-upper-lipness and didn't seem right, but I did, in front of the wig lady. She asked if I'd thought of a shorter style. I was trying to tell her that I did have a lovely short cut before... But I didn't let the cry out properly and stuffed it back down like I've been doing for years because I thought it was right and didn't want to be a nuisance. Afterwards I went to the toilet specifically to cry, but it just made my headache worse and I thought sod that. Then 'hello' I realised the new chemo has turned my wee bright red!

Later… Baby Girl has pharyngytis – running a temperature of 40 degrees for 48 hours. Life doesn't stop because you have cancer... the boiler still breaks, the TV breaks, you still experience road rage, narky checkout girls, can't find a cleaner, kids still get sick, people are still who they've always been... little boys still squirt perfume in their eye at 6.50am.

For people whose cancers haven't been removed, you could easily convince yourself that the effects of chemo is the cancer killing you. That you're dying. How many times have you said/thought that on a hangover? Thinking about the future makes me sad. Partly because nothing else matters at the moment – I'm existing in a status quo where nothing that mattered matters but then... *nothing* actually matters, we just think it does. That kind of philosophising doesn't last very long! My brain can't cope!

I am purposely not making a list of all the things that hurt. My thumbs feel awesome, so do my ears. My feet are beautiful, eyes gorgeous, shoulders magnificent. My wrists are delicate, my chin is cute. My nails are beautifully shaped. My heart beats strong and evenly. I have chosen to be in a daze through this round. To switch off and not really be here. Like my labour with my daughter. And it made it much easier. Deep breathing escapism. The 'chemo brain' helps to slip into a meditative state. I am now the Queen of Meditation! This is getting rough but I'm glad it is. You can't sail through chemo – you can make the best of it but if you don't have to dig deep, what's the point? Without eyelashes, some make-up has scratched my inner eyelid – exquisite pain! With that, mouth ulcers and a cold / chest infection, I have felt in the grip of it but today I've had a word with myself. It is in fact just those things. It's just a cold, it's not cancer, it's not chemo, it's just feeling rotten. It's happened before, it'll happen again. I *am* healing. There are some good days on chemo, like, *almost* normal days, it's not *all* hard. The skin around all of my orifices is starting to suffer – just delicate, tender, easy to damage. I get jumps, twitches in my legs towards the end of a cycle. How am I still finding my long hair everywhere? Seriously?

Next chemo session - where I dropped a tablet worth £85 on the floor. Yikes! This time I remembered to take the bandage off the cannula site before the kids got home. Nusband's got Man Flu. Help!

December 2012

I get so pleased every time I have a poo! It feels like a personal achievement. Constipation is a much-cited side-effect of chemo but I'm keeping it at bay.

How chemo is different to what I thought:

I thought 'attacking every cell' in my body would hurt. It doesn't. I thought that if I got a cut or a mouth ulcer, it wouldn't heal and that by the end I'd be covered in sores. No, heals fine.

Last week's chest infection reminded me what it's *really* like to feel ill. Coughing causes back muscles to ache, painful sinuses, pressure headache – that hurts! This is tiredness, nausea, a dopey feeling. Hard to remember what I've just done. But on my fourth round, coping is getting easier not harder. Just have to get plenty of rest. I don't sleep well, I think due to the steroids but I work a lot with my energy and being relaxed – it helps.

For the most part I am the first person the kids see in the morning – which always lifts me – and the last person at night. It's important to me that they have that. That's my priority.

On chemo everything is dry. No bogeys or ear wax. The metallic taste in my mouth and the smell of me have become normal. I need to be careful of projecting symptoms. Last week I was convinced my nails were falling off and my eyelids were sore. Both were just badly placed cuts. I try and gee up my positivity and make a list of 'Reasons to be Thankful. I manage 23 things.

In other news what I'm finding re: treatments is that (a) It doesn't seem to be getting worse. In fact I can learn / predict how to manage the symptoms better as time goes on and (b) no two rounds are quite the same. There will always be a difficult day, but not for the same reason – this time it has been a chronic sore throat – again with the pain! I thought we'd established this. I don't like pain!

When it's hard to cope, I keep reminding myself, nothing lasts long. I find if I can deal with it in moments, no moment is too hard, or if it is, it is just a moment and then that moment is gone and I'm one moment closer to being done. I'm seeing a new Oncologist today, to decide my fate. I know I still have some *Titanium* left in me but I'm not sure how much. I must have slept ten hours in the last week.

What's great about feeling awful is feeling better. That everyday feeling that we just fritter away on life, never giving it a second thought. Clearing away the tissues, cleansing in the shower. The fog lifting, the grip loosening, surrendering to my body – letting it surf the wave rather than paddle against it. But sometimes I can't get up. I can lie in a cold bath without the energy or momentum to get out.

I've had a Eureka moment! Four weeks now I've had a nose that drips like a tap! I have kept thinking, when will this cold ever end? But it was weird, it stopped responding to the nose spray and didn't affect me in bed at all. Then it hit me. I found Nusband, threw my head back and asked: 'Do I have hairy nostrils?'.

After some consideration, he decided 'Erm, no'. So, it's not that I'm ill. I just have nothing to stop the snot from falling out of my head! It literally *is* like a turned-on tap! So glamorous! Have you ever stopped to think how valuable your nose hairs are? Nope, neither had I!

My skin is crepey it's *so* dry. I drop things a lot. I was told this was to do with lack of grip caused by the chemo – not sure. I don't drop heavy things (like children) but lighter things all the blummin' time... This round has been very emotional. It's been a rough ride but these few days of feeling normalish have been bliss. Something to look forward to.

Nusband's just said...

'Steriods working?'

'Why'

'You're singing S Club... in bed... at 11pm'

'Oh yeah, I guess.'

I remove my serenading self from his embrace and say...

'You're tired.'

'You're wired!'

Around this time, I run into a previous client of mine, Cathy, I've not seen her for years, since I stopped business to have the kids. We bump into each other at the entrance to Tesco. As soon as our eyes meet we both know. I raise my hat and she raises her scarf to reveal our bald heads. We discover we were diagnosed almost at the same time. Both breast cancer but not the same kind. We exchanged notes and going forward seemed to keep bumping into each other. She's a powerhouse! Out every day, walking when I can't get myself off the sofa. I see her powering past, through the window! Sometimes I can get to her before she's zipped off again. This is completely normal by the way, we had different cancers, different chemo drugs to fight it and we're different people. I remember reading about a guy in the states still working a 60-hour week on chemo. Knock yourself out fella, I'll be staying here on my sofa, not cleaning the house.

My oncologist has reduced eight rounds to seven. The last one will be the 25th January. That's next month! Will be here soon! The nurses had to try four times to get the cannula in my arm. I can only use one arm as my right one doesn't have enough lymph nodes left to shift the drug, so my left arm veins are overused and shot. They keep popping and bulging under the skin... delicate little things.

Have considered harvesting some hairy caterpillars for my nostrils. It was the first time since that first day that I'd spoken to my neighbours at chemo. They were both solid Scousers, funny, friendly. They were both dying. We chatted about all our kids, about Christmas, about a new grandchild due in July. I said, 'It'll fly'. On reflection, probably not what he wanted to hear. I'm crying now. Everyone's tough in the chemo suite.

I went to my sister's 40th birthday. Got my wig stuck in a chandelier – otherwise pulled it off well... the party, not the wig. My other sister's wife, Hannah (you'll meet her later), she styled my wig, kept apologising for pulling my hair - lol. Nusband and I danced *Gangnam Style* – only spoke to people about cancer. Left at 10.30pm.

The fog came down the next day. How this drug is different... My trumps don't smell so bad but my mouth is worse – a horrible taste, a sticky film covering my mouth and tongue, like I've eaten ten bags of Haribo, lips like I've eaten salty crisps – numb. Tired. So tired. I ache deep in my body, my spine. Kidneys. Stomach. I keep eating hoping to hit the spot but can't. Can't taste anything. My nails hurt, feel fragile. When I get food stuck in my mouth I can't get it out with my nails or tongue!

The other day I went to an electronics shop to pick up a new phone cover. I asked the manager if he could help me find the right one, save me looking. He took me over to the shelf and pointed out the one I wanted. I picked it up but of course I dropped it. It landed on the floor between us. Both of us bent down to pick it up. Our heads almost met. As they did, my nose released an enormous mucus bungy, stretched the distance to the floor but didn't spring back. Nope, just pooled between us. We looked at each other. I said nothing. Literally nothing. What is there to say? 'I'm so sorry my mucus has stopped staying in my head. You see I have no nose hair…' I picked up the phone case, paid and left. Say your prayers to the Nose Hair Gods people.

Losing my eyebrows, eyelashes. How much worse? Then I remember that's not how to do this. Don't engage with it Em. Stand back and watch the experience flow past like a river. I do some relaxation exercises to help and achieve an almost comatose state and flatly don't accept fear. All worries are fear. Tell them 'OUT!' Must float. Can't think about the lonely journey. The life I'm missing.

I am very short with the kids on my tired days. I fear causing irreparable damage. I had an especially bad morning yesterday when I seemed to repeat myself constantly and they just ignored me. So so frustrating. Sometimes I find it hard even just resting near them. Their physicality, their noise, lack of understanding. I find it all too much and have to take myself away. I have to be able to dip into and out of conversations but the kids, being kids, demand my attention.

I got very dramatic on Thursday. I let myself get very scared about when I'll start to feel better on this round. Because it was taking a bit longer. I convinced myself that the drug was burning me from the inside out – what a vision! This is because it accounted for a lot of my pain. Tingling fingertips, numb mouth and lips, what I was calling 'rectal burns' and the aches in my stomach and gut.

Then I remembered I had actually burnt my finger on a lighter and the constipation that is now a regular houseguest had caused an abrasion, but look what hysteria my mind had imagined! Enough with the melodrama. I felt a lot better the next day.

I'm finding it hard to write due to the loss of sensation in my fingers. My fingernails are so sore! Any pressure put on them or using my fingers is tender. If I catch them on something, a tiny bash, it's soooooo painful! Things I can't do because of it:

- Do up small buttons
- Open tangerines
- Take the price stickers off Christmas presents
- Open tissue boxes
- Get chewing gum out of the packet.

I'm trying not to think of them coming off, which can be a side-effect of chemo.

Christmas Day, all went well, good excuse to wear a Santa hat. I had to cut open all my Christmas presents with scissors as my fingers don't work, but had a nap and a dream about Patrick Swayze – a gift to myself! I had ordered every Christmas present from the sofa, had memorised my card details. A good day was had by all.

January 2013

It is really hard to recall short-term memories while I'm like this. I've just thought of something but it's gone. My skin started peeling off my hand today. The palm side of my fingers. I'm pale. I forget that, then I look in the mirror. I look ill but feel ok. I don't have just dark circles around my eyes, they're sort of purply red.

Chemo day is not a bad day. You wait around – the worst that can happen is that they don't find a vein first time – or third! But the nurses are lovely. I point to a burn I got on my hand on Christmas Eve, off the oven. It had healed before new year. I asked my nurse if that meant the chemo wasn't working? She looked me in the eyes and smiled 'No, that's not what it means'.

Remembered that thing I couldn't remember – eyelashes. Fair enough they have to drop out but they don't drop out they drop in! I can't taste food – so unsatisfying to just experience the texture of food with no taste. Just tastes of chemicals. It's not that this feels bad, just that it feels unfamiliar. Don't assume it's pain, horror, anguish. A lot of it is just different. Yes parts of it are rubbish but not all and I can cope with small bits being uncomfortable, unfamiliar – break it down – tiny steps.

So in the grip of this drug – this is how it feels. Different parts of my body ache for short periods. This is the 'deep bone ache' I was warned of. It aches like losing weight or like I walked up Snowdon yesterday. It can be in my nose and my rib cage, then in my spine and my knee. It's not too bad or too long anywhere. My skin is soft, nails are tender. I can feel the pulse in my gums – itchy neck. Worst part by far is the gross taste in my mouth. 'Lack of taste sensation'.

This is not worse than the common cold. First round comes with fear which I think makes it worse. Not had any pain killers so far this round. Have had heartburn/constipation medicines. There's a lot to be said for not losing one's nerve! Falling for the hype of what you imagine is happening / what people tell you/ what you see on TV. I feel anxious about life after chemo but think it's just the waiting to see what will happen. I want a big change. We'll see. People have said that part is hard. I can see why.

I look my worst. No eyelashes – ashen pallor – plucked turkey – but feeling good. Makes no sense. Still need to take it slow. I'm trying not to have too high an expectation of my body at this time – I've recovered so well from this round. I've been expecting more from myself in the second week but have had to concede. I'm having chemo, still tired. It's OK to feel uneasy, bit rubbish, unsure.

I had my last treatment on Friday – needed to temper my elation in the Oncology Dept. – not everyone was feeling chipper. Had last steroids yesterday – 8mg dexamethasone x2 a day. Last injection.

I'm raring to go, workwise, in my head. But I couldn't even if I wanted to. No rush. I'm physically tired but not mentally. Lips hurt like they're dehydrated. Awful taste (sharp) in my mouth. Can't move. Wake up exhausted. Ache like muscle ache. Not in bad spirits. Last time now... This isn't brave, inspiring or impressive. It's my life – if it was you, this would be your life too.

So my last chemo is slowly filtering out of me. It makes my trumps smell like metallic brie. 'I love the smell of chemo in the morning...!' Not.

I'm still finding my hair in places you wouldn't expect – clothes mostly. In fact contrary to what the scare-mongers said, I think my resilience to chemo increased as time went on. It shocked my body initially but it seems used to it now.

Years later, there would still be parts of chemo that I miss. Mainly stepping out of life and responsibility.

The diaries you have just read form part of my talk for chemo nurses that I present now at the hospital that cared for me. It is titled: *The Emotional Effect of Chemo or Service User Experiences of Chemo.*

Every time I do it, I am reminded of the staggering resilience of this bunch of skin and bones. I remember what my body went through, seven times! How it gathered up and knitted itself back together every time. That I could sleep and it would heal me. That most of the time, it performs that dynamic job constantly, without us really knowing about it. Mind-boggling! My relationship with my body shifted like an earthquake. My body isn't something to be lambasted with criticism. It gave me my most precious gifts – my babies and more time with my family (that I am now keenly aware, not everyone gets), feeling well again, giving me potential and opportunity. It is my most valuable asset. Most valuable. I won't look at it in distaste again. It's an outrage that this is what it took to connect me back to my body.

This period also provided me with some important lessons. The opportunity to really stop and tune in with myself, with my body. To notice and be more conscious of how it feels to be in it. To read and explore and learn more about how it works and how it is linked to what we think, believe and feel emotionally. It also taught me that I LOVE FOOD! God I love it. I now know that food is such a source of satisfaction for me. Joy even. A life without being able to taste food is like a beach without the sea. What actually is the point? It gave me an opportunity to reflect on the simplistic narrative we create around food restrictions and diets. As if simply stopping food is that easy. It totally isn't. Food is a primal need, a source of immense comfort, satisfaction, fun, joy, tradition, community, togetherness. Not just as we package it, a reward for exercise. Somehow in the wellbeing conversation, most links to pleasure and its value have been erased. But my relationship with food was yet to undergo another gear change, and not in a good way…

Age 35

My treatment was over. I remember reading something that warned me I might feel adrift when active treatment ended. That my lifeline had been cut. I didn't really feel that. I felt excited about it being over, no more shleps to the hospital, for a start. But also time to move on. What I wasn't expecting… was not being *able* to move on. Mentally, physically, emotionally. I hadn't realised this is where the real work would start!

Firstly I want to talk about hormones. You remember I had mine paused, all periods stopped while I was having treatment, with an implant directly into my belly every month. It was fine until… Holy cow they came raging back. Until this point hormones for me were something a bit jokey, a label we slap on girls and women – often a euphemism relating to being bitchy or hard work. A throw-away comment and not really taken too seriously. In fact as women we often reject and repress the idea that it's hormones impacting our behaviour because so often they're cited as reason for our outraged behaviour, behaviour often outraged in the face of female inequality, no less - so I feel a bit of a traitor in what I'm about to say. Let me tell you hormones and the onslaught of them are serious. Nusband reflects: 'It was like a freight train had hit the house', I knew I was doing it and I felt so out of control, powerless to it. As an adult woman, basically going through puberty, it was flipping horrendous! But it also gave me a new perspective on teenagers going through the exact same thing but without the perspective to see what it was, instead it's something that has just crept up on them. Of course you'd believe it was actually you! Not chemicals!

The next thing that happened was, you remember, I'd been keeping my feelings in a jam jar in my stomach, well somehow, the jam jar opened! I say this for the benefit of cancer survivors and their loved ones - take care of your patients after the storm. For you, perhaps the worst part of the journey is over, your friend or loved one has hair and energy and is back to doing all the things they used to do. Except, they are probably still tired. Probably still running into walls they're trying desperately to smash down in the name of normality. I remember hearing Katie Perry's *Roar* for the first time and thinking, *Yes! This is my new Fight Song*! And then quickly realising I was still only really at *Meow*.

Those loved ones of yours, now the dust has settled, might just be starting to grieve. The point of the jam jar was to protect myself. My body compartmentalised all my emotions in favour of coping with the day-to-day of surviving cancer. Once the threat had passed, I now had chance to start sifting through my feelings and… it wasn't pretty! Speaking of fight songs my new one became *Diamonds* by Rhianna. It was a reminder of the opportunity that I'd been given but also of all the support I'd had through my friends and family. They 'shone bright'. And the nature of the song made it easier for me to cry. Sometimes you just need a song but it wasn't just a bitter sweet feeling I had.

They say the process of grief involves – denial, anger, bargaining, depression and acceptance. The denial thing I'd done pretty well. Now I was on to the anger phase and boy was I angry. *So* angry. And the person who kept getting it was Mum. I knew I was doing it, I kept apologising for it but then lurching into it again. She just held it for me and listened. I remember saying it didn't make any sense – it felt pretty irrational.

And over time, it got better. And although I didn't see it, it was congealing and morphing into bargaining. Throughout my recovery, I had read a lot, learned a lot, theorised a lot, *spent* a lot on trying to avoid getting cancer again. I learnt what to eat and what not to eat. What products to use in the shower, in the make-up bag, around the home. I learnt not to use perfume anymore, tampons anymore. Not to drink alcohol anymore, not to eat sugar anymore, to use only organic products at home and work, to juice, to exercise, to meditate, to take my vitamins all in a form of bargaining but also as a form of power. To regain some of my own control over my body. I was amazed how, being motivated by something other than the way my body looked, put a really different spin on my relationship with it. I was *for* it, totally in support of it. The thing is, and I absolutely didn't see it at the time, it was making me incredibly miserable and probably quite difficult to live with. I would feel awkward visiting friends with my new 'regime'. I made sure I wasn't too demanding with my needs and would eat and drink what I was given, but then would feel disappointed in myself that I couldn't live the way I wanted to (needed to) for my welfare. I'd open birthday and Christmas presents of bathroom bits that weren't paraben-free and have to arrange my face to show false appreciation. It felt like constant conflict, a tug of war. As a life, it wasn't sustainable for me on many levels.

Firstly it could only ever exist in bouts, there would always be an event, a holiday, a party, that would break the routine. I thought I wasn't invested enough to forego the celebration and communal ritual of food and drink. Yet most of the time I was pretty strict with myself so if I did have a blow-out, the toxins would hit me hard. I'm just not a do-it-by-halves kind of person I guess. I was mostly purist then occasionally would fall off the wagon. I was controlling, conflicted and I was obsessing.

The second reason it's not sustainable is because that schedule of idealised 'wellbeing' activities is a job. It's not trying to raise a four and six-year-old, hold down a steady job, while making a family meal-plan or cleaning the odd toilet on the side. If every bit of food is a transaction, a weighing up, logged and monitored – It. Is. Work. As an aside, unless it *is* your job or your highly paid job relies on your body (giving you a deep personal motivation), then maybe it's doable (and bear this in mind, next time you're absorbing life advice on social media – if it's their full-time job, they don't also have… a job to try and fit in on top of it), but for the rest of us, we can hope to do maybe one of those things. If you *are* fitting all that into your life, you're benefitting from some sort of privilege in there, even if it's just the privilege of time.

Which brings me onto the third thing that makes it unsustainable – the cost! I consider myself pretty privileged but wow! This life, it's not for everybody. Do you know how much organic wax strips are? Or that you can't buy them here, have to get them shipped from The States. Or how much organic massage oil eats out of your take-home profits? At the root of it is big bucks! Out of your pocket, into someone else's.

Health, weight-loss, wellbeing are often packaged as one of our base needs, what we need to survive. And it does involve food, so it can be a bit confusing. If we look at Maslow's hierarchy of needs, in fact it's not at the bottom with food and shelter but right at the top in 'self-actualisation'[25]. It is what we are able to attend to, once *everything else* has been taken care of. If there's actually any bandwidth left over. It's not essential, it is a luxury.

However, sustain it I did, or at least I tried to, oscillating between feeling pride and failure. Restrict and rebel. It wasn't until much later someone introduced me to orthorexia - an eating disorder disguised as 'wellness'. Somehow, having been packaged totally differently for me, I hadn't realised it was…oh blimey! It was a diet! Or that it was messing with my mental health and that my feelings about food and my physical health were pretty messed up too!

I remember explaining my new 'anti-cancer' protocols and a friend gently pointing out to me, 'But cancer just happens'. Remember 'healthism' which puts us at the centre of, and responsible for, our own health? I was so steeped in the *belief*, and there's plenty of content out there to back up this mindset, that I must have got something wrong - that I could fix it. At the time, I refused to believe my friend, to accept that health just *is*. It may be a manifestation of the life you lead but also it may not. 'Healthism' for some, might not be that 'healthy' after all.

There were times along the way, I noticed that something was a-miss. When I went to turn down my daughter's first batch of self-made cookies! Seriously four years old. *Just eat the flipping biscuit dude!* And then again on a holiday and after a significant batch of sugar-free time, I had a glass of wine with Nusband. Woke up feeling like I'd been at the Bad Mom's wrap party. I want to be able to enjoy a glass of wine with my Nusband! I want those joys in life but they made me feel like a failure. I remember tussling with the idea that a life spent like this, might not actually be worth it, for a few extra years they might give me!

This is in real time now 2021 – I recently found a photo of me, from around 2015 and again it makes me question if I had an eating disorder. I don't recognise the picture. I'm standing on my sister's balcony in Tenerife. I look thin. The thinnest me. Not underweight but I can see it's not me. It wasn't healthy knowing me and what's normal for my life. I ask Nusband if I had an eating disorder? He said no, I always had it under control, 'and you had been very ill.' It's just… I'm not sure it was illness-related but fear of the illness returning. I concluded, not an eating disorder but disordered eating. I can never unknow the rules of what I now see as a food disorder (in its purist execution), but I can de-escalate them in my routines and while it didn't threaten my life, I could see how a disordered pattern of eating can really set up shop in our minds. Positioning people's comments as jealously or ignorance on their behalf, rather than concern.

So we've covered denial and bargaining, next was depression. Every year, September would come around and I'd get scanxiety with my mammogram for my remaining boob. And every little thing was cancer, from a broken nail to a stomach-ache. What did I attribute these things to before cancer? I had no idea. And frustration, definitely a big tick there. So ready was I to get out into the world and crack on with life and life kept cracking me back on the bum! I'd start having alarming thoughts like, is this what it's always going to be like? Will I *ever* feel normal again? But to explore the depression, we need to re-wind to 2008…

After The Boy One was born, as often happens, one of the hardest things was a sense of losing myself. My identity shifted and I didn't know which way I was headed. I decided I needed something just for me, so I enquired about starting ice skating lessons. It was just what I needed, they had a creche for the little man and I got a couple of hours a week to focus on me. It's something I'd wanted to do since childhood, and it felt great to get my badges (sewed them onto my jumper like an absolute dork) and certificates. I was so proud of myself! However, it wasn't to last long, my pregnancy with The Girl One being just around the corner. But it didn't deter me and as soon as she was old enough to go to the creche too, I re-joined. On my return I got to know a new skater in my group, Trista. She was in her fifties and our skill levels matched. Although she was a lot steadier and more precise where I was a bit more, throw myself around, we were often paired together. Before long, we were good friends, often using the free skating time after lessons to chat and meeting up for a cuppa. I was struggling with The Girl One not sleeping and Trista loved catching up with us, gave me sage advice and had a soft spot for my girl.

The timelines are a bit muddled in my mind, but it was probably 2011, when Trista told me she'd been to see her chiropodist and he'd expressed concern about a mole on her heel. Later she told me the doctor was worried, then the consultant. 'I've always worshipped the sun and it was an area I just never thought to put sun block on.' When she told me she had skin cancer, I had to make a decision, am I in for this? Having watched my Dad handle it, I knew it was a commitment and I knew I was scared about not just witnessing it again but the commitment you give to support someone with this journey. It was a momentary decision and came out as a yes…

It was an odd conversation when I had to tell Trista that I had cancer too. It's a weird thing to bond over, but I guess it brought us closer. We'd meet up and swap notes. We spent a day at the beach, with a picnic. She visited me during chemo.

When Trista's cancer came back, probably 2014, things weren't the same and I had a feeling I knew why. Or perhaps we'd just drifted. My only experience at that time of a relapse had been my Dad and that didn't work out so well. Then, one evening, my phone rang, I looked at it 'Trista Mob' flashed up on the screen.

'Trista!'

'Oh… no… sorry, is this Emi?' My heart sank. It was Trista's husband, telling me what I'd already suspected and letting me know when the funeral was. I got off the phone and found Nusband. I cried and cried, I was hysterical even. In front of the kids, it just came so seemingly out of the blue and for once I could access my real emotions, immediately.

The following month, we had a holiday booked. I remember sitting on the beach staring out at the sea and crying silently. It had hit me so hard but also, it had hit me when I finally had access to my emotions again and I was feeling them all. For Trista yes, but also for myself, for us, what we'd been through. It was cathartic and necessary and a period I knew I just had to endure. I was starting to understand that about losing people. You can't rush the process. I was also still angry. I was angry that she hadn't told me, that I didn't get the chance to say goodbye. It was such an irrational emotion and deep down I understood it. If you're dying, your world must shrink to just your most special people, to honour that time with your nearest and dearest, not a random from the ice rink! And with time the anger went too. I have happy/sad memories of us. The irony is, at diagnosis I avoided making friends in support groups through the hospital, other women like me, because I couldn't face losing anyone else and I lost her anyway. I didn't go back to the ice rink for five years. I'm crying now… think I'll leave it there today.

Age 36 - Picking Life Up Again

I returned to hands-on body therapies around two years after my diagnosis. I discovered a new massage system a bit randomly on LinkedIn. One of my contacts was moving to America with a British product and I got in touch to find out more. The product was called Hydrotherm and sounded A-mazing. It is basically a warm waterbed massage system. I have no idea why I'd never heard of it, much less experienced it. It had been a while since I'd done any new training for my actual job as a body therapist but the time felt right. I trained, I dallied with the idea of becoming a trainer for them but decided it wasn't the route I wanted to take and I set up shop again. I hadn't done hands-on therapies since The Boy One's waters had broken and The Boy One now lived in the room I used to do it in. For around six months I did mobile therapies. This involved setting up at each new home, including filling and lugging around the two enormous water bags. I loved the treatment, the benefits were obvious, allowing total muscle relaxation and what's termed 3D massage. Also great, incidentally for anyone having undergone breast surgery, as you can do a back massage all face up! I didn't love the continual set up.

It was while visiting one of my previous clients, Kate that she told me that her friend, Diane was setting up a local tea rooms. It was going to be in a shop that had been vacant in the village for ages. The property was huge, with three floors, a proper Tardis! And

Diane was wondering what she could do with the room upstairs. It would become my work home for the foreseeable and the ladies downstairs, my work family. I had no concept of it at the time, but this move was a life-saver for me. No schlepping water bags round anymore, my job became 40% less work and I just love being there. I would credit Diane for playing a pivotal role in my recovery but she's too won't accept that so I'll just leave it here. I don't think it's too wide off the mark to say she is and has created the heart of the village and the atmosphere is gorgeous (On reading this, one of my first readers added: Amen!). Just walking through the door makes me smile, even on tough days. As a team – there's thirteen of us - we all get on, we socialise, holiday together. I've never worked in a team that works, it was a revelation to me that work can be so easy-going and so much fun. This seemingly insignificant comment from Kate, which lead to an introduction, might have lead to my most important career move. In addition, I love my job, honestly there are worse things you can do with a life than make people feel good and yourself relax all day! Life is good at The Old Bank Tea Rooms!

I started to see more and more clients who were coming to terms with a cancer diagnosis. My longtime client Cathy started coming back to see me. I especially loved helping these clients to feel better. It made me want to complete The Christie Hospital's *Diploma in Adapting Complementary Therapies for Cancer.* I found it really interesting, learning about all the different types of cancer, different types of treatments, the impact of hands-on and hands-off healing, the few apparent spontaneous recoveries. My final assignment had focussed on a critique of research about how our emotions might manifest into physical ailments. It was hard - the hardest qualification I've done.

Age 38

I attended a screening of the documentary *Embrace* at Manchester Printworks, created by Australian Body Image Champion, Taryn Brumfitt. I was with my sister and two friends. The film begins with Taryn explaining her reverse-before-and-after picture that went viral. Because it wasn't your usual – here's me fat, here's me thin inspo pic. The first image depicted Taryn at a body building competition and the second showed her, demurely naked, and looking, well… normal, real. Like a Mum. She talks candidly about the sacrifice the body building had taken on herself and her young family. The time away from them but also what it was messaging for them, particularly for her daughter. She also talked about the behind-the-scenes banter at the competition, that even though her peers were among some of the fittest, possibly on the planet, they were still wrangling with their body hang-ups. Who will be happy with their bodies? If not them, then who?

Through the documentary Taryn introduced us to a full range of inspiring women, either sharing body image issues or overcoming them. I watched the whole thing, enthralled.

As the credits rolled my mind was reeling and my eyes were leaking. I told the girls, 'I think I'm going to need a minute'.

Someone else was inside my head. At last! This is where the seed really started to grow. Where I knew I wanted to do more. A quote from Melinda Tankard Reist in the *Embrace Documentary* stuck with me: 'Why should the vested interests of advertisers come before the well-being of children and young people?'[26] When you witness something life-changing like that (and I've been witness to a few) you sort of have to hold it. Be with it. Let it sink in. Let the inner workings of our bodies shift to accommodate this new reality. I continued to go about my days, not really sure what just happened or what it meant. But slowly I realised what I had to do. With the work I had been doing with photographer, Jaine, I had created an online platform called *Mummy One Boob*, (now on Insta @TheCancerNude) it was a place where the images we were creating and the journey we were documenting lived. I went back to the gallery and started to type. Furiously getting it all down right there, the blog being my conduit for expression and before I knew it, it was done. And I realised what the whole journey with photographer Jaine was about. Not just creating a visual reference for the journey and encouragement for future cancer patients. It was for everyone. And it was about one thing, so simple. It was about a deep, satisfying, fulfilling acceptance. About reconnecting ourselves back to our bodies. I hadn't realised it but I had been falling in love with my body! No questions, no doubts. I looked in the mirror and I said 'Yep, you my friend are *for me.* You are mine and I am truly and sincerely grateful.' It was a peace-making experience and left me feeling changed. Ahhh acceptance – a love letter to my body!

A Tale of the Unexpected

I'd been trying to contact *Fashion Targets Breast Cancer* to see if my *Mummy One Boob* work could have any synergies with them but could I find an email or phone number to call on their website? Only a physical address. So I decided in all my shrinking violetness that when we went to London for my son's ninth birthday, I'd just flipping well pop in.

I left my family eating ice creams at the Tower of London and took a short walk to the office. What I discovered was not a *Fashion Targets Breast Cancer* office but a *Breast Cancer Now* office, which made sense. I walked into the glassy foyer, I took the lift and found someone to talk to. I don't think they were *Fashion Targets* necessarily but they were really keen to hear about my work with *Mummy one Boob* and all about how it's changed my relationship with my body. It was only then that I realised I was dressed head to toe in pink. I swear this was not intentional, I genuinely wear a lot of pink – it's a self-healing colour. Anyway, the lovely lady bemused at my pink getup took my details and said someone might be in touch. They might have something I could get involved with.

I went back to my family and put it to the back of my mind.

My Gratitude Diary – May 11th 2017

I am amazed and utterly grateful for the skills of my surgeons, creating me a lovely pair of hooters.

Closure

The last of four surgeries. It's funny to think, that first day in my consultant's office, the one where I had Baby Girl on my knee? I remember thinking, let's just get this dealt with as quick as we can. If it had been up to me I'd have had a double mastectomy then and there and *stich me back up and I'll be on my way.* I hadn't realised it takes time – 2017 is year five! I hadn't realised that it is a process both physically and mentally and also that recovery can be a very beautiful process, not just all the grey doom and gloom that the media would have you believe. If you live, in fact from what I understand, even if you don't, it can be pretty life-affirming! And I don't say that flippantly, having lost too many, too close to me.

My second surgery was to remove the implant that I'd had put in my remaining left boob, to try to mimic the perkiness of the replacement one on the right. It just never felt right. Too big and obtrusive. I'd look in the mirror and not see myself, my shape, even with my clothes on. I realised, maybe for the first time, that I'm attached to *my* body, that I like it the way it is, I like to recognise it like an old friend in the mirror. Don't take my shape away from me!

I wonder if anyone saves up for a boob job, goes through the build-up and comes out wondering what these weird firm balls in their chest are doing and where did my body go? But find it much harder to acknowledge in those circumstances, that it was a mistake. Of course, the opposite may also happen, they may look in the mirror and say – there you are! Where've you been all my life!

My third surgery was a fat transfer, lipofil surgery. They basically take the fat from your legs and bum and inject it over the silicon implant to make it feel, less plastic - more like normal tissue. My surgeon looked at my body, 'But you'll have to put some weight on.' This resulted in a brain fart. Weight *on*. This again challenged the 'eat clean' lifestyle I had developed and lead to yet more conflict and confusion. I settled on eating one flapjack a day from the Tea Rooms. When I say these boobs are made out of flapjacks, I'm not kidding! Almost *every* woman I told about this forced weight gain, offered me her fat instead. Another indicator that *all* women feel the need to shrink their bodies. Even the already slim ones!

And that brings us up to surgery number four. Every year I'd find another lump. Five lumps in five years. The results always came back the same: 'You just have lumpy boobs'. But every time I went down emotional rapids of worry. To a greater drop and much quicker than the first time. It was life-limiting for the time it took to receive the results. And so the decision was made to go ahead with a full bi-lateral mastectomy. This surgery came with a side-order of lipofil to boot!

By now I'd become pretty laid back about anaesthetics. There was none of the anxiety of the first time, I recognised surgeries as just a really deep sleep and when you wake up, it's done! Like magic really. Try telling me that on the first go round though!

I've just had a great memory! During lipofil - surgery three, my consultant had asked me to take my knickers off – because they get in the way. The only problem was, they were lucky knickers, a Union Jack on the back. I remember not wanting to take them off! What about my luck! Still banging on about it as I counted back from ten. Later, once I came round again, a nurse was helping me to wake up. She was laughing, telling me how I was mumbling something about my knickers as I came round! Still having the same conversation even though hours had passed!

But that's not all, on this, my fourth operation, I bounded into the operating anti-room, excited to finally be getting some closure and the ability to move on. I jumped on the bed, and asked the room, should I take my knickers off?

A male nurse turned around and said in a camp voice 'Love! We've only just met!'

I guess I ran in to that one! The atmosphere prior to this op was buoyant, joyous even!

Following the op, I had my new body - nipples totally removed, but two matching, unlumpy boobs, similar in size to my own! One still slightly bigger than the other as one had had its skin saved and one had had it stretched. Implants don't last forever, maybe ten, twenty years. But for the foreseeable, I was done. And it felt great.

As I've said there are a number of options when it comes to reconstructing your boobs, including not doing it at all. It is such a personal decision. You can have different parts of your body repurposed into boobs, thighs, tummy rolls but I already have twelve scars that required stiches (sorry eleven, one was a steristrip!) so more scarring and unknown effects of this put me off, as did the extended recovery period and the cracking of my ribcage to re-attach arteries. And yet I wasn't ready to go without, I wanted to feel as back to normal as I could, so this was the right path for me. However do know that if you find yourself in this position, you have a choice and at the end of the day it is your decision. Nobody can tell you what to do. Which is a blessing and a curse.

I had been much more indecisive about this surgery and my photographer, Jaine, sage that she is, summed it up perfectly. She said, it's like the first mastectomy, I was pushed off a high diving board into a pool. This time, I'm working up the courage to jump off myself. I've got longer to think about it, more options to consider. She was absolutely right. My heart goes out to those who also have to make that difficult choice if they have the BRCA gene. Before this, I always thought they had it easier - I never considered how hard that must be.

Gratitude Diary - June 2nd 2017

I got a casting call! From *Breast Cancer Now*! For a campaign with M&S! Very, VERY excited! Thank you!

Gratitude Diary - June 8th 2017

Thank you for my *Breast Cancer Now* casting going SUPERBLY! For lunch with The Duchess (unofficial sister). For the train service and meeting new, wonderful people. For London. For my in-laws making it possible...

This day nearly killed me! I was less than a month post op, hadn't yet made it back to work. But I just couldn't miss it. It was a casting call for this year's *Breast Cancer Now* campaign in collaboration with M&S, marking *Breast Cancer Awareness Month*. I made it down to London and back in a day. I arrived at the offices of *Grey London,* the creative agency working on the project, and right from the start I was treated like royalty. Part of the casting call involved being sized for underwear, I was then photographed in it, holding up my hands to show any visible tattoos – with my occasional exhibitionist nature, I was in my element. I was interviewed on camera. Two women sat on the other side of the camera. There was a short paragraph that we had to learn and a few questions. I don't remember them all but I remember this one.

Grey: What has cancer taught you?

I thought for a while, I wondered how to put everything I'd learnt into a sentence. The rejection of idealism, the importance of gratitude, that my body is incredible. It wasn't something I'd ever thought or verbalised but it was just right for the moment and just came out.

Me: Cancer taught me… I am enough.

I wasn't expecting it and I don't think the interviewer was either. She welled up, so did I. The casting finished soon after. As I stood to leave I turned, put my hand on the doorknob and heard the faint whisper. 'Yes.' I was sure I'd heard it. I didn't like to hope or think of it as a guarantee but I couldn't help feeling a fizz of excitement powering on my fatigue as I made my way back to Euston Station.

The Boobie Shower – June 2017

It was around this time that I decided to celebrate my end of treatment with a party and what else can one do following a double mastectomy, than throw a Boobie Shower. I invited all the girls from the Tea Rooms and we had such a laugh. I wore a T Shirt with basic boobs drawn on the outside. We had boobie sweets, boobie games, some nice food and drink and generally a jolly old time. The perfect way to celebrate a new beginning and an end to surgeries.

Gratitude Diary - July 7th 2017

I got in! *Breast Cancer Now* wants me! Can't quite get my head round winning something. It's going to be AMAZING fun. Who knows where it goes?

Gratitude Diary – July 24th 2017

An amazing day meeting the *Breast Cancer Now* and M&S team and all the other girls doing the campaign. Everyone's lovely.

Gratitude Diary – July 25th 2017

A photo shoot at Big Sky Studios. Thank you. I did well, a great shot came out of it. Made some great contacts.

This was another full-on day. Shot just ten weeks after a double mastectomy, you would never know from the images. It was a weird day. In hair and make up for hours and with our underwear styled (tit tape), it felt weird being the centre of attention. I was also conscious that this day could lead somewhere for the rest of my work. It also reminded me how much we use body shame or self-criticism to ease the wheels of friendship. I felt getting to know the other girls on the shoot wasn't helped by me not engaging in body-criticism. The night before, at the hotel I had discovered another amazing documentary about body image, *The Illusionists*. I watched the whole thing on my phone! I remember talking about it and the *Embrace* film and it creating puzzled faces. I felt it would have been so much easier (less challenging) to just stick to the trad narrative of body hate, and bond through that.

I had had experience modelling with Jaine of course and she made me feel so at ease. Here the crew was huge. I feel I will have come off as cocky, it felt like playing a role of a confident model. The images are testament to that but the nerves! I put them in my belly jar and just got on with it. I came away happy that I'd done a good job but not sure I'd ingratiated myself to anyone.

I was so excited to see the backdrop, it was a beautiful candy pink. From behind the camera the crew gave me some direction. They asked me to dance. There were people everywhere watching me. Why had I suddenly forgotten how to dance? What kind of dance? I know I stiffly moved my body, I have no idea what it looked like 'cos I was completely overthinking it. The lights were bright, two massive wind machines turned on and eventually I let myself go a bit. And just like that it was done. We did some more group shots which also came out fabulously.

I saw my final image. It was awesome. It caught my awkward dance really well lol.

Gratitude Diary – August 10th 2017

Just more days like this please. A day of filming / collaborating on the M&S shoot. Felt so proud, really supported and accepted. Thank you :0)

The shoot location was a large and beautiful Victorian terraced house. The top floor was taken over with hair, make-up and changing. I later found out the basement was where the creative team were getting rushes of the filming that was taking place in the middle two floors. We were creating a short film for social media, that would accompany our campaign and it would be based on the answers we gave at the casting.

We first did a piece to camera, where I said 'Know that you are enough, exactly as you are.' I remember I had a water bottle up the back of my bra as I'd lost weight since the casting #realitycheck!

I don't know whether they asked or I offered but it became known that I'd be happy to be naked. Everything was handled so beautifully with the common goal of raising awareness, yes for breast cancer but I also had a separate advantage of being entirely at ease in my own skin and proud to show off what it has been through. I felt and still feel no shame. The crew this time was smaller. My job was to undress from my underwear, get into a bath and immerse myself under the water.

I was completely naked. The end result was that you see me slip off my bra, you got a glimpse of my scarred breast and a beautiful shot of me, my, then purple, hair, disappearing under the water. These are cut together with all of the other girl's gorgeous pieces, later you see my head come out of the water, smooth down my hair, wipe my face with my hands. The end-product was really moving. It's there on my Insta if you want to go looking for it (@BodEquality).

Unbeknownst to me, the rest of the crew was downstairs watching the rushes as they came in. There was a vibe of: Will she? Won't she? And squeals when I did. To this day I couldn't be prouder of that work. Along with the other girls, we created something really special that day.

Gratitude Diary – 22nd September 2017

Saw the M&S films today for the first time. WOW! They are magical! Thank you!

Breast Cancer Awareness Month

Gratitude Diary – 2nd October 2017

The AMAZING Breast Cancer Now / M&S campaign. Having good new friends. Thank you!

When days just stopped feeling real. We were taken to the M&S flagship store at Marble Arch and as we approached, there we are. At least eight feet tall in the window, on Oxford Street! The campaign for *Breast Cancer Awareness Month* centred around M&S donating 20% of the profits of a selection of bras to *Breast Cancer Now*. In store there was more branding with us on. Posters big and small. I am so proud that it created a truly diverse series of images in a landscape where I'd never seen that done before. We were on cloud nine! Social media was lit up with the campaign and there was a piece about us in the *Daily Mail* and on the M&S website. All I could do was watch and wait to see if any of the links MummyOneBoob.com would take off.

The following day I took the bus to Knightsbridge. I remember pointing out of the bus window as we sailed past *us* on the high street. I even squealed to myself 'It's me!'. The passenger in front must have thought I was crazy.

On my facebook page there are people, friends old and new, posting pictures of themselves with 'me' in M&S all over the country!

Gratitude Diary – October 10th 2017

What a day! Appeared on *Loose Women*! Got what I needed to say out. Got a free cashmere jumper! Got a great positive response. £80 in my Mummy One Boob donations account. Met Dawn French. Great day. Happy. Thank you, thank you, thank you!

A day headed to The London Studios but first to an apartment above the Marble Arch store to be fitted with M&S clothes. There was a rail of clothes all ready for us. I tried a few things on but they just didn't seem to be right. They weren't me. Our contact asked if I'd seen anything I liked. Actually the other day I had seen a really cute jumper with bright stars on it. I didn't know it was cashmere. I didn't know it was probably one of the most expensive items in the shop! The contact sent someone to pick one up and brought it back with a pair of jeans. As I stepped into the jeans it irked me that 'super skinny' was emblazoned on the inside of the waistband but when I got them on, they fitted so nicely. With the jumper too I felt much more me. They're still my favourite jeans.

Of course I was nervous. Of course I put my foot in it. This campaign happens every year or two and I knew some of the last campaign's girls were with us in the audience. I also knew the presenters would be coming to me for a comment. When we arrived I recognised, sitting behind us, some of the girls from *Breast Cancer Now's* social media. Our group was excited and buoyant to be there. I excitedly said 'Hi! Are you the last ones?' to which I got a somewhat mumbled reply.

I later re-watched the previous campaign, called The Last One, the closing scene is:

'I won't be the last one to die of breast cancer, but there will be a last.' I believe all of the women sat behind me in the studio had terminal cancer.

I had a good idea what I wanted to say but as time wore on my mind kept oscillating between focus and poise and 'How the heck did I get here? What am I going to say? What am I doing? Why were those girls unfriendly?' I would have it together then completely lose my train of thought. Dawn French was interviewed alongside the panel and I loved that she talked about *always* being asked about her weight and her weight loss and how it doesn't define her. Frustrated that that's what is always the focus for her. Although here we were talking about it…

Later they came to me:

Loose Women: Now Emi, you say doing this shoot that you did, it completely changed your attitude to your body. In what way?
Me: Well, the cancer itself completely changed my feelings with my body. I write a blog called Mummy One Boob and throughout the various stages it has documented how my body looks and I've just got such a new-found respect for my body. We are so quick to be fixated with what our bodies *aren't* and what we *can't* achieve with our bodies. We don't spend nearly enough time thinking what we've *achieved*, what talents we have, what we've accomplished, the children we've created, the races we've won, the amazing battles we've fought *and won*. It's just completely changed how I feel and I just want to share it. (Throughout Nadia Sawalha was smiling and nodding).

I felt like I nailed it. I know I went on to pay gratitude to M&S and my co-campaigners but I just wish I could remove those two words 'and won'. In the film you can see the woman's eyes behind me drop as I said it.

I've never been one to toe the line and it was a total ambition move for all the right reasons. The truth is, it *wasn't* M&S that gave me confidence (although that would have been a sweet line for them) and I never said that it was. I'm not about to contribute to making up corporate marketing nonsense – and they never asked me to. Perhaps the question was a mistake in production. But of course I do feel badly for anyone currently battling cancer. In my work as a body therapist I regularly treat those with a terminal diagnosis, *I* had a diagnosis, my Dad died of cancer, Trista. It is not a subject that I feel in any way flippant about. I just feel it also has so much to teach us, if we let it. We are all here for a limited time. I also had a duty to all the hard work I'd already done. It did up my Insta followers (you can find the interview on there @BodEquality) and upped donations to my site too. Neither were great shakes, a little, not a lot. Maybe some people were annoyed and maybe no one was. I spoke my truth and I stand by it.

After my interview on *Loose Women*, still sitting in the studio, something shifted. I hadn't practiced what I said, it flowed out of my total conviction, my passion. I realised that I had voiced, probably for the first time, my life's purpose and the feeling was overwhelming - otherworldly and a bit numb, like birthing a child! I realised it would take an extraordinary amount of work and today was Day One of God knows how many days… years.

I returned home, to my life, my work but the frenzy going on around me was still very much there. Social media was still full of friends going to M&S to take pictures of themselves with my picture. I couldn't sustain my energy and excitement to match that of everyone I saw who wanted to congratulate me, it was exhausting! A stranger stopped me in the street and told me I'd 'done the village proud'. It was lovely but equally I felt exposed, a sense of hyper self-awareness and pressure for this all to mean something, to leverage the opportunity for good but I had no idea how.

Also in the months following my fourth and last op, I was on a mission to get the weight off that I'd put on, still not seeing the irony or contradiction in this. Thirty days of almost no sugar, turned into ninety days, turned into half a year. Like I've said, I couldn't see that my insecurity had been bought again, but this time, it wasn't in the name of the perfect body, but instead in the name of life expectancy, survival. I developed a fictional lump in my throat, every test under the sun was done with no explanation. My lips would go numb. I kept rejecting the diagnosis of anxiety... Eventually I realised I was having a sustained or series of panic attacks. How do celebrities cope with this?

It was, as it usually is, a family holiday that broke the cycle, it's harder to control what you're eating away from home. A trip to Tenerife and a well-earned break after the M&S campaign. I made peace with what had been going on inside me. I decided to believe (because we can do that – we create our own realities) that the stress would kill me before the sugar. And that's where I've landed, with still a nod to maintaining a healthy lifestyle, and never again feeling like I'm denying myself of the things I want.

Once the dust had settled on the campaign I began to start thinking more productively. I had been working on my second kid's book, I had self-published *Pants Hats*, a picture book to raise money for *KidsCan* a children's cancer research charity, back in 2015. Singer Emma Lanford and Producer Mousse T even re-recorded their *Think It's Cos I'm Cool* song to my new lyrics, to go along with it (YouTube if you want to see). I was now working on my second. I want to briefly jump back to 2015...

We were on holiday and I was heavy into learning to juggle. The Boy One was telling me how his Headmaster could juggle. He was watching me and I started to sing / trumpet the circus theme... 'Da da daddle addle ad da daa da…' and out of nowhere, The Boy One started singing… 'Don't go knocking at the circus door…' to the tune.

I said, 'Where did you get that from?' He said he just made it up.

'Are you sure?'

'Yes!'

I felt sure it must be something he'd heard at school or on kid's TV or something. I googled it and nothing came back. For the rest of the holiday I kept hearing it in my head and messing around with different words to go along with it. By the end of the holiday I'd written another kid's book, this time inspired by The Boy One (Pants Hats had been The Girl One's idea), so that felt right. The story, a sing-a-long set to the circus theme (*Enter the Gladiators - Thunder and Blazes*, if you're wondering) was all about inclusion and self-esteem and difference. It centred around a mermaid finding her place in a circus.

When I got home, I contacted my two good friends and we set up a creative team. Amy on design, Lisa on illustrations and myself as writer. We treat it very much as a hobby, something to do in our spare time. But fast forward two years following the brilliant diverse campaign I'd just been involved in and I realised it could be so much more than what it was. I didn't want a fictional mermaid, I wanted real, diverse people, addressing the real issue of body difference, gender roles, finding your purpose, anxiety and shyness to share your talent and passion. The girls were really good taking the news of basically 'I'm so sorry but all that work we've done needs to go in the bin, can we start again?' And that's what we did. *Don't Go Knocking on the Circus Door*, would eventually launch in 2021! Showcasing real body diversity for kids. But still, there was more I could do.

Age 39

All of my fears about the cancer impacting our sex life were unfounded. This in no small part because Nusband's gaze never faltered. My boobs are fairly firm, often cold and numb, having had the nerve endings cut during surgery, so it can sometimes feel a bit weird, but only really if I let it, which I don't. They don't at all feel like boobs and it wasn't a free boob job. If I allowed myself to, I *could* miss my soft, comfortable, Mummy boobs, but what's the point? They're not coming back. My biggest concern had been that I wouldn't be able to feel hugs anymore. That I couldn't have a satisfying hug with my babies, my friends, my Nusband. In fact it's nothing and now (four years later) it never enters my mind. You hug with more than just your boobs of course! You hug with your arms, shoulders, neck, head, heart…

I had been quite happy without nipples. What's a nipple between friends? Between lovers. Not much as it turns out! Then one day, an online friend tagged me in a post. A tattooist from Keighley was looking for bodies to practice areola (nipple) tattoos on. She had put me forward and I got it! I'd seen areola tattoos on Instagram, I followed STACIE RAE A.R.T. (Areola Restoration Tattoo) online but knew she was in The States and I wasn't about to fly out for some new nips! I thought the ones I'd seen looked pretty good and definitely lifelike with a 3D effect. I'd even had Stacie send me some press on tattoos of them and I'd tried them out. My consultant hadn't realised it was me in the picture with them on!

I arrived at the studio and met Lucy, who heads up the Nipple Innovation Project, a charity helping women feel empowered and dignified following a mastectomy. I was excited but also nervous. I'd had a tattoo years ago at Uni, it was tiny and I remember it being agony to have done! I hoped they would be kinder here and give me some pain relief. Then just as I was about to go through to start the tattoo, another woman arrived, she had an American accent. It took me ages to figure it out, you probably have already. It was only Stacie Rae! I told her 'It's Emi… Mummy One Boob?' (as I was then). She remembered me. I couldn't believe it, I was only going to have my nipples done by Stacie and Lucy! Even more excited now but also tattoos still hurt. There is no magic cream to make them not. Well there is, but you have to break the skin for it to work, so it's sort of not really a pain free route. But… I was brave and stuck it out. I remember looking in the mirror afterwards and just feeling… complete! I hadn't thought I'd needed it, but it was closure! And my little twist? You'll have to check my Insta lol @thecancernude!

I had to go back to have a top up a few weeks later but then with just a month to go before I was due to get married, I have my nipples back. It's in silly things like catching sight of myself in the mirror and there not being something missing. It's looking passable as normal. It's not important but also I was surprised what a difference it made to me. Lucy is an incredible advocate and source of support for women like me, post mastectomy. Her *Nipple Innovation Project* is definitely worth a look, if you ever find yourself in the market for new nipples!

Age 41 - What of Health

So there we are, we're almost at the end of my body story. I have two years left until I am classed as being in full remission. But I'm not stuck anymore, and it feels great. I'm happy and I have a great relationship with my body. I'm not wishing for a body I'll never have. Not steeped in fear of eating a banana (the sugar!) Don't come to me asking what works for me habit or foodwise, sure as eggs is eggs, it won't work for you, because we're all different, living different lives, in different bodies with different interests and passions – more on that in a mo.

What I can say has helped though, is acceptance. An easing off of resistance to my body. A decision to look at it a different way. Glances in the mirror that spark nice thoughts not awful ones. A compassion that just wasn't there before, a respect and loyalty.

Without our bodies we are nothing.

We have nothing, there is nothing, well none of this anyway. Our bodies contain more cells in them than stars in the galaxy (that we know about) and they perform many thousands of functions to enable us to live and live well. They constantly strive for health, regardless of how we treat them. I love this great passage from Bill Bryson's *The Body: A Guide for Occupants:*

"Top trauma surgeon Ben Ollivere reminds us that 'Most of the best technology that exists on Earth is right here inside us. And everybody takes it completely for granted.'" [27]

Having sustained a serious illness I can vouch for that. It does it all so effortlessly… until it doesn't. When we're reminded of its constant work to keep us alive and well. It's a total privilege. Which when we think of some of the norms around how we behave and think about our bodies, the judging and criticism, we can come off more than a little… misinformed.

There was no good reason why I got cancer. The odds are so low – just 2.7% of new cancers falling into my age bracket. I was young, not overweight, not a smoker, didn't drink excessively, it makes no sense. Same for my dad and the odds of losing him at such an early age to a non-smoking, lung cancer. The odds of me miscarrying four times that of the general odds – two in four, not one in eight, according to NHS statistics. The odds of my waters breaking early less than 3%. My body has had the odds stacked against it and yet, here it still is, here we all are. It is strong. It is resilient. It has achieved and created the most wonderful things, jobs, relationships, home, people! And do you know the most beautiful thing about it, the thing I am the most grateful for? I bet you don't give yours a second thought. My body's biggest asset is… its energy. Its ability to get up and do it all again. To get up and do it with gusto. That I can rely on a power that now is always there when I want it. It is an absolute gift. That's what I love most about my body.

Well done bodies for allowing us to live our lives, do our jobs. For stamina, energy, function… for dealing with trauma in the coolest, most nonchalant sort of way, just quietly gathering itself up and bringing itself back together. We could be thinking SO differently about our bodies…

The Science of Diverse Bodies

Why we are Not all the Same

We relate our bodies to food and food to our bodies without a whole world of context that is also part of the conversation...

Here's a tempting overgeneralisation. There is only one type of body. All other bodies are the one type with varying layers of fat on them. One valid body, one healthy body. Underneath, everyone has the same basic make-up that responds the same way to the same conditions. Tempting. And overgeneralised.

This is a chapter about, what I'm going to call *Body Intelligence* – like emotional intelligence but for bodies. It is going to highlight the many, many, *many* ways that our bodies are all different. It might challenge your understanding of how the world works and your concepts of diet and weight loss and I apologise for that because I know you (and your feelings of hope) might be fairly invested in them. I came to a lot of this information feeling *How is it possible for this to be true? Surely I would know if this were the case? Surely someone would have told me*? However, as you will see, much of this is actual science or common sense.

Genetics

When I was younger I remember reading an article indicating that some people are genetically predisposed to being fat. Just once, in my entire life of reading magazines and content about bodies. At the time, I remember considering: *Is it an excuse fat people use to justify being fat, not getting fit? Must be some kind of hoax. The world wouldn't,* couldn't *be organised the way it is or present the landscape of bodies that it does, if this were true... could it? Would it not constitute the biggest case of false advertising, misrepresentation*? But as I found out, actually, not an excuse. Science.

And as I've already touched on, science isn't a commercial force, it's a force of discovering the truth, but sadly people don't always generate much money out of selling the truth. You can't shave your legs with it, eat it, drive it, curl with it (bend it maybe). It just is. If you want it, you need to go looking for it. Which you have, so pats on the back for us. But *that* is why we don't already have this information in our brains, not only does it not generate money, having this information deep in our core beliefs would even give you pause to spend money on other things, impacting things like a media outlets' advertising revenue (This is the entire basis of the documentary *The Illusionists* and it's fascinating – you can watch it right now, on the internet). So content like, 'There Are Fat Genes', has been silenced through the usual media outlets. Like many *real* aspects of bodies, it has been buried in favour of more lucrative content, resulting in a totally skewed version of bodies.

In fact bio-medical scientist, Dr Stephen O'Rahilly of Cambridge University who by the way, acknowledges 25 different genetic anomalies linked to obesity[28], explains: 'When we studied the children carrying these gene mutations, they weren't predominantly becoming obese because they weren't burning off calories, they were predominately becoming obese because they ate too much. They had a profound appetite drive, they were not satiated by the same amount of food as their siblings carrying the normal genes.' [29] I've just sighed. It's a lot to take in. Some people just *do* still feel hungry, starving even, yet the food those people are eating may still be healthy (mind blown). More on this in a sec.

But there is another problem, just like anti-fat bias (fatphobia) exists in all aspects of our culture, it also exists in the world of science. Much of what I'm going to share with you wasn't championed by science from the inside either. The overriding assumption that fatness is behavioural and controllable, being too strong and ultimately unchallenged for many decades.

Metabolism

Now for an inconvenient truth… Your body may never change. There is significant evidence that it won't. Most diets don't work. Or maybe how we approach bodies and diets, is causing this number to be so large. In his book *The Truth About Fat*, Anthony Warner ably highlights how a very small variation in our natural basal metabolic rate can predetermine our weight. Variable metabolic rates are rarely a consideration in modern convos around diets, weight loss, health. Usually because someone is trying to sell us something to 'fix' us. But real they are and their impact can have huge results as Warner explains: 'A hardly perceptible five per cent shift, easily possible given known genetic variations among people – would have led me to gain several kilograms of excess body fat every year' This would be despite there being no difference in his eating habits.[30]

In fact, our metabolisms work hard to protect our natural weights, I want to back this up with a very scientific study of me and my dog Phoebe. Phoebe is a Malinoise cross. A Malinoise is a Belgian Shepherd - a relative to the German Shepard and she likes to run. She can run and run and run and… you get it. I went from a fairly active body therapist to a two-hours-of-walks-a-day dog-owner and my body changed. My body fat reduced. My muscles got stronger. I was thinner! However within a few months, I noticed a drop in my energy, had started to feel a bit rubbish and tired - I could feel it in me and you know how I hate to feel energetically drained. I started to eat more to get my energy back up and didn't think much of it but here I am now, back where I was. Body corrected itself. But not just for me this metabolic voodoo. A year into our adoption of Phoebe, we decided to put her on a raw meat diet as it helps to calm some dogs down (questionable) and the next time I took her to the vets, she'd lost half a kilo! Slightly worrying as there's nothing of her anyway. Sure enough, we kept an eye on her and up she is back to her previous weight within months. Phoebe is doing really well and we're both learning more about how to behave!

This story reminds me of one I read about a husky dog sledder in Alaska who had noticed peculiarities in eating habits of her dog team. Blair Braverman writes on her Instagram 'Some of them eat thousands of calories a day and are still complete string beans. They eat literally three times as much food as everyone else. Some of them can eat, like, a tablespoon of kibble, and the next day they need a bigger harness. They're easy keepers; their bodies naturally want to be bigger. Which is good! Easy keepers make great sled dogs.'[31]

And maybe your body does that. And maybe no one has ever explained the many scientific roots of physical diversity not just being about us accepting everyone, *even* if they're fat, but that some people *will* be fat. It's normal. It's natural. It's how we're designed.

What I don't want to happen here is to put anyone off pursuing healthy goals. No way! But if you're someone who has been a long-time rider on the weight-loss carousel, and never seen a lasting improvement, maybe we need to have a word. A life spent outside of the idealised image of how a body *should* be, is not a wasted life, the waste is how much attention we pay to it. A life spent hankering after something so physically out of our reach as to be impossible -

is a loss. A total waste. And remember at least 95% of us that fall into that category.

Health is another question. Pursuing health is well worth doing but be prepared the results may not look the way you (have been programmed to) expect them to. I'd bet my bottom quid most diets are abandoned because the dieter has not seen the superficial physical transformation they were looking for and gives up, seeing no other reason to continue. As an aside, from a cancer survivor, let me tell you, if death comes knocking early, you're gonna feel like a shmuck with that kind of ankle-deep thinking. Health *is* possible, but health isn't a purist removal of all sugary/fat foods. And actually, with enough life-shiftery, losing some weight *is* possible. Writing in the Huffington Post, Daniel Bartlett has this to say:

'Losing weight in the short term is very simple and any good tactics will get you there but losing weight in the long term is strategic and needs consideration of the psychological, the physiological and the biochemical.

An integrated strategy can flip the 90% of failures to 90% of successes but is too complex a message to become mainstream. It needs too much preparation and hard work.'[32]

All I'm saying is, your body may never change. And that's OK It's got to be, because otherwise we're going to continue wasting our valuable lives chasing something we'll never achieve.

Hormones

How else can I convince you? Let's talk about leptin. What is leptin and how could it be impacting our body shape and size? With research spanning back to the 1960s but crystallised by Professor Jeffrey Friedman of Rockerfeller University in 1994 (still more than 25 years ago), it has been found that we possess a gene – a hormone to be precise - called leptin and it controls our appetite[33]. Biologically, in all of us, our fat stores send messages to our hypothalamus to let it know that we are full. More fat cells create more leptin and our appetite reduces. The opposite also happens as fat cells start to be used up. Hello diet days, fun times! As our fat stores reduce, our appetite *increases* and the battle begins.

(As an aside, what this does mean though is that for most of us, our bodies, when left alone, have a fairly natty way of maintaining their natural weight. We don't leave it alone though.)

What's more, some of us, through a quirk of genetics don't create leptin – I can hear your gasp from here – I know right! Others of us, don't have the receptors to detect for leptin. I know - it's like boom! My brain had to rearrange a tidge to accept this info:

What so, it really isn't fat people's fault, or at least might not be, or at least we can't know if it is or it isn't so let's stop pretending that weight loss is for everyone?

Yes body shape is physiological and in some cases, completely beyond our control. Yep, some people don't have the triggers in their body to let them know that actually one tub of Ben and Jerry's is enough. Some people continue to crave food as if feeling starved at the point that others would be popping their waistbands.

Another Awkward Conversation

I want to ditch this science and take you back again to my teenage years. I could never understand why I would get in trouble if ever I asked Mum about her body. If I asked about her not walking the dog, when that was the *reason* we got a dog. Or if she ever thought about dieting, or being healthier. I'd get into trouble and I could never make sense of it. Mum would blow up, the conversation would be shut down. I can't even remember how, I can't offer you a conversational soundbite. I just grew to know that was a subject we don't go near.

Then recently I had a client, a new client. They had started on a new healthy plan and had started to see their success. It was as a result of being diagnosed with Type 2 diabetes. This diagnoses they said, really focussed their mind on getting healthier. We talked for a long time about our bodies and it developed into a really candid conversation. I explained the background of my work and that I passionately care about campaigning for all body types to be valued. I had a theory and thought this would be a good place to find out if I was right. I gently asked if they thought that sometimes, when a person is very overweight, a sort of disconnection happens. I guess a bit like that day for me back in high school where I learnt I had the wrong legs, but on a much greater scale. I wondered then, when the body has become a source of: shame, disappointment, self-criticism, judgement, ridicule, trauma, if some people compartmentalise it. Deny its existence almost. Of course they live with it, but also separate, reject and deny it. Maybe it is also linked to a feeling of utter helplessness.

It was such an awkward conversation, but the signals I was getting were all positive. The client confirmed, yes that was just right. They said that six months previously, we *couldn't* have had this conversation. They weren't in the headspace to acknowledge it. What a *cost* to someone's mental health. What a loss. The client also said 'It's so nice to hear someone be on our side. You just assume *everyone* is looking at you and judging you.' Heart-breaking.

The fat people this affects have taken ownership of the problem, they too judge and criticise themselves, and see it as their fault and their self-esteem is often on the floor, when it really isn't as simple as all that. Fat people have internalised shame, it's possibly why this problem is still such a big problem, we, the world, and *they* often believe it's their fault. Unlike other discriminations such as racism or sexism, fatism doesn't have a groundswell of outraged righteous victims (although fat advocacy is thankfully growing). Historically, victims feel ashamed, isolated and internalise the abuse. When as we're learning it often isn't their fault and the solution we've been trying to use, won't work.

In addition, the separation of body and soul, body and mind, is a real barrier to finding our authentic health. A disconnection that I won't pretend to understand but a severing of ourselves to our bodies on a much more extreme scale. It's wrapped up in not being able to exercise for fear of judgement, in weight-cycling through periods of restriction and rebellion, of jibes and jeers leading to self-loathing. Of hopelessness and pointlessness and a sense of disempowerment to change any of it so just eat the Goddam cake! It is trauma.

And… it explains why I used to get into so much trouble. In Mum's defence, you may not be surprised to learn, I was not an easy teenager, nor the compliant third child she was surely hoping for! In my defence, I believe the way this played out robbed us both of her self-agency and confidence. On showing Mum this piece she replied simply 'At last somebody understands'. But there was more to understand. Let's go back even further, not in my life but in the life of someone I loved very much.

Body Stories
Aunty Aileen

'Aileen! Are you talking? Do you think it's ok to interrupt this class?'

'Erm…no Sir, sorry Sir.'
'Well maybe this will remind you, I want silence in this classroom. Now, Aileen stand please.'
Aileen stood up.
'Now get onto your chair.'
Aileen slowly stepped up onto her chair.
'Now onto the table.' Aileen looked around and back to the teacher. She paused and then took another step, up onto the desk.
'Now class let's all have a good look at Aileen's bandy legs?' He let her stand there in shame, with all eyes of the class on her. I don't know the reaction of the class, or how long she had to do it. It's a second-hand memory through Mum.

Mum: It was Aileen (Mum's sister) who was first diagnosed with hypochondroplasia. Her doctor had flagged up a potential problem of having short limbs. Wanted to send her for checks to make sure her pelvis could support a pregnancy, luckily the answer was yes. When she did get pregnant, she attended an ultrasound appointment. The Sonographer silent in their work, seemed to take too long. 'I'm so sorry Aileen… I can't see any arms or legs on your baby'.

Fearing the worst, that her baby would have her condition or perhaps a worse embodiment of it, an X ray was organised and an agonising wait. Once the Xray was done, she was told she'd need to wait another two weeks for the results. 'Is there no way you can give me the results today?'

'I'm afraid not, these X Rays will need to be assessed and sent to your doctor.'

Aileen left the Radiology Department in tears but soon, a nurse caught up with her. 'I'm sorry, I know I shouldn't do this. Your baby is fine. It has its limbs.' Aileen must have been wrung out with relief.

Mum: Then, after your cousins were born, Aileen found herself back in the hospital for a routine operation. Finding it hard to get up onto the couch, the doctor asked, 'Do you know anything about your condition?'

'No, just that I have short limbs.'

'Do you have children?'

'Yes.'

'Are they… the same?'

'No, I'm happy to say, they aren't.'

'Would you like to know more? We have a geneticist here in the hospital. I'd be happy to refer you.'

Mum: He confirmed that Aileen had hypochondroplasia, a form of short-limbed dwarfism. What this means is the bones of our arms and legs stop growing but our muscles don't. The reason Aunty Aileen's legs curved outwards was because just one of the two lower leg bones continued to grow. I have the muscles of a 5'7' woman squashed into a 4'9' frame. (Mum reminds me she was 4'9' and a half – that half was always important. She's 4'7' now.)

Aileen asked about the rest of her family, why didn't her children have this? The answer was, it can get passed down but it gets diluted with each generation (hello mega calves). If the father is tall it's less likely. The geneticist enquired about her siblings and asked to see Mum and her brother. This confirmed that their generation of the family did indeed all have hypochondroplasia.

Mum: But my body, my trunk is normal height. Sitting down I'm as tall as anyone else. I remember being put in the front row for a school photograph because I was short and my teacher asking 'Are you sitting on your satchel?'

My Mum was late thirties when she received her diagnosis. She tells me that Aileen's young exposure to body shame left her with a lifetime mission to prove her worth, to show people she was good enough.

I was devastated when we lost Aileen in 2019 to cancer. Some days it still doesn't feel real. My body still hasn't caught up with it as I think about calling her.

The Science of Diverse Bodies Continued…

I don't mean to harp on about my mega calves but I discovered more…I recently found out that a cousin on my father's side had had his DNA tested and the results showed we have Nordic ancestry – where Viking mega-calves were all the rage! I'd say it's quite rare for someone like me to have so much information about the genetic fabric of my body. Only serendipity has lead me to these discoveries. Who knows what genetic secrets our bodies hold! Shall we start dialling back the shame now?

Skeletal Ratio

This is something that relates to my family especially but also to everyone. I had never really considered it and it was YouTube yoga teacher Flo Niedhammer who brought it to my attention. As soon as she said it, I realised to was actually just common sense. In describing The Child's Pose Flo highlights: 'So for most of you, you can probably reach your forehead closer to the ground but for me if you can tell in the video, I have very long legs and a very short torso so for me my child's pose is just with my chin resting on my knees. So the purpose of me telling you that is that you can already see and check for yourself that each body is proportionately designed a little bit differently depending on your skeletal structure. This pose might look different to you as it is for me and that's really one of the first lessons of yoga, we're not trying to mould or conform our bodies into any specific shape. Each pose is done 7 billion different ways and your body is one of them.'[34]

Trauma

Another reason we are all different, and maybe hardest to look at is found in research that strongly links childhood trauma to obesity. Sexual abuse or ACEs – Adverse Childhood Experiences – which can range from toxic stress to parental suicide. This is a conclusion historically reached by many researchers and corroborated with Swedish research in 2014. The Karolinska Institutet undertook a meta-analysis of previous studies, looking at a sample of 112,000 participants[35]. While of course, not being the only causal link, it *cannot* be overlooked. It is estimated by the Centres for Disease Control and Prevention that 'More than six million obese and morbidly obese people are likely to have suffered physical, sexual and/or verbal abuse during their childhoods, according to the CDC's ongoing ACE Study.'[36] The causes behind this can be that: the trauma has created a food addiction and psychological comfort; that some sufferers want to desexualise their bodies and feel safer that way and also that trauma in the critical developmental stages of a child's life can impact their neurobiology making them less responsive to rewards. Ready for more? It's ok to take a break if this is hitting you hard.

Socio-Economics

Science also tells us that body shape is determined by our socio-economic standing. The British Medical Journal in 2017 asserts that 'people with lower socioeconomic resources, both as children and adults, are more likely to have a higher BMI and increased risk of obesity in adulthood.'[37] BMI aside (in the world of fat advocacy, the BMI scale is much dismissed as arbitrary, problematic and not fit for purpose… and I agree), the findings still stand. Poorer people are more likely to be fat. Also, The Glitch, causes fatter people to be more frequently overlooked at job interviews / progression so you can also argue that fat people are more likely to be poorer[38]. Sigh.

Privilege

This touches slightly on another aspect of body shape in that it talks about privilege. It's true that some people live more completely in The Glitch than others. If you're still struggling with the idea that everything I'm saying is real, that surely you just eat less, move more and lose weight, there's another factor that might be playing out for you and that's your thin privilege. If you find maintaining a low weight is within your grasp, and so assume everyone would, you're talking through a screen of bias that maybe you can't see. As Aubrey Gordon writes when talking about anti-fatness in thin people: 'They believe that they've *chosen* their body'[39]. Not just economic privilege but also physical privilege. Thin privilege. It's like white privilege, but for thin people. Of course looking at why some people might be fat, also brings into question why some people might be thin, that's just as important in the conversation about the natural diversity of bodies.

Even though I don't feel particularly thin, I still benefit from thin privilege. It doesn't mean that I necessarily *feel* at an advantage, and yet I still am. The world is organised for people like me. Theatre and airline seats, restaurant booths, turnstiles designed for people like me. High Street clothes sizes range for people like me, the generalised way we talk about bodies, generated for people like me. Assumptions that almost everyone has about bodies, have them based on people like me.

What's more, at the extreme end of the thin privilege scale... If you are a gym bunny, drinking matcha, making almond milk for fun, then let's not forget the privilege of your resources. The time, learning, equipment, energy, life choices, are not afforded to everyone and the fact they might have been born that way, their body make up and genetics might put thinness within their grasp in a way that it doesn't for other people, making it *way* easier. Let me give you an example. During lockdown we had themed food weeks and for one week we decided to cut out refined sugar. To make all the goodies to replace refined sugar cost me no less than £50. It also took my knowledge of what to make, where to find the ingredients in the supermarket and all of it could have been avoided if instead I'd spent £5 in the confectionary aisle. It's all privilege. It's my privilege. And is another reason why we are all different.

This manifests itself in seemingly innocent ways. Ohhh heck, I hate using this next reference. I have a book, I'm reading it right now. It's a gorgeous book that I have loved so much that as soon as I finished it, I started it again. I chose it because I've been reading and audio-booking so much intense research types of books for this book, I wanted total escapism, total light relief. It is the story *Olive, Mabel and Me* by Andrew Cotter. You will have probably seen one of his lockdown memes on the socials where sports commentator Cotter shifts his focus onto the antics of his two gorgeous Labradors, hilarious, adorable. My Phoebe Dog is a Labrador cross so I feel even more connected to his writing. I can't express enough, how much I love this book and don't want to tear him down (buy the book folks!) But… on page 121 in trying to understand why some Labs are chunkier, he mentions a study. In 2016, Cambridge University discovered a genetic glitch in 23 per cent of Labradors that meant messages were not being passed to the brain that they were full (leptin? Possibly). However on the very next page he remarks, about fat dogs 'But it's really not that difficult. Feed them less or exercise them more.'[40] It's the over-used and simplified version of calories in/calories out that we've all been programmed to believe. Even in the face of his own research about genetics, he couldn't swerve that traditional trope about bodies.

Oh Andrew. Please know the pain it took for me to use that example. But it is a perfect one, of the ubiquitous nature of thin privilege, the damage it can cause (more on that later) but it also highlights… it's not Andrew's fault. Because of The Glitch. Whilst I haven't had the opportunity to explore this with him directly (but would love to – call me Andrew!) it is a pretty fair working assumption that he most likely doesn't even know he's done it. He is unlikely to have been trained in body intelligence (most of us haven't). He's grown up with The Glitch too, and from what I have seen he lives in a thin-privileged, active body, so that would suggest that he has no reason to question The Glitch. The Glitch appears to be true - like trickery. But also poor, fat, hungry dogs.

To be clear, I'm not a crazed fan of overfeeding dogs, my dog would literally eat ALL of the things. If there was an Oscar for procuring food off plates using just your soulful eyes and a well-timed whimper, she'd be right up there. AND she's never offered me any of her food, not once! Although she's quick to point out, I've never licked *her* face. But not even in a cute, funny tale about two dogs can we escape the tyranny of The Glitch and our iron-clad (simplistic) belief in fantasy bodies and how to get them. Actually, it is hard. And sometimes impossible.

If all of this does feel a bit challenging, it's OK, that's quite natural but it is in fact good for us as Brain Researcher Lisa Feldman Barrett points out: 'Exposing yourself to stuff you don't know and maybe even ideas you don't like, might make you feel crappy in the moment but actually it's a really good investment'[41] she's talking here about brain flexibility which makes us better problem solvers.

Mind Health

"My daughter's lucky, she's anorexic."
Splash, 1984

While we're here talking about privilege, in *Watching the English,* Anthropologist, Kate Fox notes that in the process of ensuring our kids have their five fruit and veg a day, and quit the junk, we may be unwittingly ignoring the food cancel culture of teens, especially in our upper classes where pseudo 'intolerances' and the latest food fads and trends are masquerading as borderline (or worse) eating disorders.[42]

Fox makes a valid and serious point. Eating disorders are the mental health issue with the biggest mortality rate. And the rate of eating disorders is on a steep incline with patients only getting younger and yet socially we are giving this very little focus and lack understanding around it. An eating disorder is a serious mental illness that can be characterised by auditory hallucinations and again a serious body disconnection. Why the steep increase in recent times? Not in small part because of The Glitch and the general public's belief in fantasy bodies (research to come). The lack of body intelligence and lack of ready visualisation of real bodies in the world around us. I'd like to point out here two further and *even more* unseen problems. Firstly that many eating disorders go unrecognised. Our understanding, awareness and maybe even recognition of BED or Binge Eating Disorder, in ourselves and others, being so low. So often the visual of eating disorders is linked to skeletal forms, ribs, spines, which brings me on to the second hidden eating disorder – anorexia and bulimia in fat people. Still a mental health disorder, still full of control, anxiety, conflict and very much life-limiting, still a loss, but still not recognised, normalised, or deserving of treatment in the medical world where referrals and hospitalisation are linked to extremely low BMIs. Dietland does not account for these people. Does not worry about these people, The Glitch *does not care* about these people. And it gives us another reason why we are all different.

Things just got really serious here and before we move on, I want to address another serious aspect of The Glitch that needs our attention. Women are usually centred in this conversation, however the repercussions of men having low self-esteem, self-worth, self-dissatisfaction, can come with more devastating effects. A man dies by suicide every 90 minutes in the UK. It is the biggest killer of men under 50. In fact all suicide is on the rise - it's the biggest killer of all young people and those with eating disorders have a much increased risk.[43]

Ben Akers is a film-maker who created the documentary *Steve* following the tragic loss of his childhood friend. It is such a moving and powerful watch (www.stevedocumentary.com). What it brings home is how important it is for men to put aside toxic ideas around masculinity and start talking and as a result Ben has developed Talk Club a talking movement for men (www.WeTalkClub.com). Akers interviewed many men from all walks of life to try and better understand why we are losing so many men to suicide. The following comes from Ben's interview with John Barry, Co-Founder of the Male Psychology Network:

"We've done some research looking at the impact of thinking around traditional gender roles and suicidality. What we found was, the more that men and women thought that they needed to be a fighter or a winner in life, the more that they thought that they had to be top dog and very competitive, the more their thinking was suicidal. When you frame things in "I must", "I ought to" or "I have to", you automatically put yourself under much more pressure than you need to. One of the other things we found in our study was that the more people thought that they had to control their feelings, the more suicidal their thinking tended to be. Within psychology there's almost a male gender blindness, we seem to have a bit of a blind spot for when men are having problems. When women are having problems, we can see it quite clearly, men will tend to want to control our feelings and when we have a problem – we want to fix the problem, we don't want to talk about our feelings we want to fix the problem. We might *really need* to talk about our feelings but it's not the first thing that we're going to try to do. They don't go to therapy, they don't seek help as much as women do, even when they *really, really* need to get that help, they don't seek it. And we had to look at these gender differences so that we can do something practical to try and solve these issues."[44]

I followed up this conversation myself with Barry, he mentioned in relation to body image that 'men sometimes genuinely don't recognise that they have an eating disorder because they think of this as something that only impacts women. This is an issue that is easily overlooked when it comes to understand male help-seeking.'

A really good text on this subject can be found in Christopher Eccleston's *I Love the Bones of You* [45], his memoir and personal account of anorexia.

It doesn't take a genius to realise that impossibly high standards of living might be impacting this devastating state of affairs and that how we feel about and in our bodies, is a factor. I talked earlier about The Glitch taking our lives, either in small ways, by stealing our life's quality, or in big ways by stealing our life… all together. I meant it. We have no idea what is going on internally for anyone other than us. It's another reason that we are all different.

Life Changes

Here's another tempting over-generalisation: the ideal body image is achievable *and* static. Like there's a 'forever body'. The truth is, from the day we are born we are deteriorating. Bumps, scratches, scars, viruses, pocks, spots, wrinkles, ops, hair loss… are visual clarity of our time on Earth. There is no standing still in our bodies. Our bodies will sweep on regardless… One day, your future self, will covet what you currently see in the mirror.

Our bodies cycle through different stages that are rooted in our biology yet are invisible in the fantasy world of bodies. What's more these cycles are not only magical (clever human-making skills) but differ in each of us. Puberty can arrive at eight years old for some and 14 for others and it massively impacts our body shape with the development of muscle and reproductive organs.

Similarly, one of the reasons we put weight on as we enter the menopause is to regulate oestrogen levels in order to better serve our bodies, improving: bone density, the brain, nervous and cardiovascular systems, skin elasticity and it can even offset some of the classic symptoms of menopause.[46] Women can hit the menopause as young as their 30's and it can last in some into their 60's. Men can tend to lose weight as testosterone levels drop (around 55) and women too in later life may see a natural dip in their weight.

What Else?

Beyond science there are also common-sense reasons for diverse bodies. How our lives are arranged, for one, what dependants we have, what else is capturing our attention. How about injuries and disabilities and how they might impact how our bodies are? Some obvious visual ones and some completely hidden. Even something as simple as people having differing interests might reflect that in their bodies. Someone with a love of running is going to have a different body to the person who loves to crochet, who again might have a different body to the foodie who loves to try new recipes and cook for others. And I support these people because I'm fairly useless in the kitchen and they help me put delicious food in my belly. *So just change your interests, lose weight. Stop doing what you love, start doing… something else.* Why? It would be a personal loss. Everyone has different interests and preferences. Say if someone doesn't like the beach or can't stand cauliflower or even nails down a blackboard. It's the same thing. We don't attach a moral judgement to other interests or preferences, or lack of. But not liking fitness, exercise, working out, hitting the gym or restricting your food intake is not a flipping crime right? It's totally normal. Isn't it? For us all to like and dislike different things. There's no law that says we all have to love that stuff. So there's another good reason we're all different. Or are we activity dictators?

What about pleasure. Pleasure plays a very minimal role in the story of our wellbeing, when in fact, I'd argue it should have a starring role. So often restriction and forced exercise regimes don't hold pleasure at their core. Pleasure, doing what we want to do, are called to do, rather than feel we *have* to do, without recrimination, should not feel like a transgression. If we frame these pleasures as infractions, where does that leave our mindset, our wellbeing?

Another reason, habits. The way we relate to our bodies and our food. Maybe you're someone who doesn't have a cuppa without a biscuit. Maybe the end of the day is signalled by a glass of wine. Maybe you don't eat breakfast. Maybe you have to walk a dog. Maybe you think, *so just change*. And people *could* change their habits, (which may not necessarily change their bodies in the long term). But also, have you ever stopped to think where habits have come from. Food habits can be programmed into us at our critical developmental age, by people who are not even us. Sometimes they are deeply rooted in connecting us to comfort - which serves a really important job in terms of our mental health.

Sometimes habits are not even rooted in *our* lifetimes. I'm talking here about ancestral programming. How you think and feel (in general but also) about food, might not be *your* thoughts at all! But may have been forged generations ago, during wars or famines and passed down as gospel. Things like, don't leave any food on your plate, or no dessert without clearing your plate, or TV snacks or simply the habit of having sugar in your drink. Diets are based on changing habits but habits are not always easy, possible or beneficial to change. It's estimated that the success rate of diets is between one and three per cent[47].

Body Stories
Bev Carter

I'm eleven stone lighter than I used to be, I have the side by side, 'before and after' photographs and the compulsory 'standing in one leg of my old trousers' picture. I share my 'weight loss story' and I now work in the fitness industry supporting people to achieve their fitness and weight loss goals; yet I also claim to be a supporter of body positivity.

At my largest (UK dress size 24, over 20 stone) my body ached, my feet hurt, I lacked energy, I felt uncomfortable, when I exercised I could only work with a small range of motion and I frequently got injured. I don't accept that being massively overweight was what was best for me, not because I'm 'fat shaming' but because for me it wasn't mentally or physically healthy. Pre weight loss, I was overloading with sugar, eating until my stomach hurt, in a way that was out of control. Now, I have a healthier body and I no longer try to use food to meet the wrong needs. It's been seven years since I reached my initial weight loss goal and people are always asking me what my 'secret' is; ideally they want me to tell them a quick fix solution, or handover an exact, fail-safe diet and exercise plan. The truth is that I don't have a secret, just lots of very complicated thoughts and self-learning.

For those who have never battled with their body; fat loss can be condensed to a simple equation of 'burn off more calories than you consume'. Except, many of us know that in reality, there is absolutely nothing simple about it. For the whole time I was overweight, I wanted to be 'thin' more than anything (perhaps this was part of the problem). For years I lost weight and then would find myself piling it back on; I hated my body and was drowning my shame with food, so the cycle would continue. My first step to lasting change, was to start to love the exact body I had and not the one that I wanted. My mind needed to be transformed before I could make any lasting difference to my physical health. Of course, 'how' I did this is very hard to explain. I think the closest I can come is that I had some kind of spiritual awakening, for me this was rooted in my Christian faith and I'd express it as a deep awareness that I'm a beloved Child of God. To people who are not religious this might sound unreachable but I'm convinced that this realisation can be found in each of us. It's discovering that child-like acceptance of who you are, your own sense of beauty and intrinsic worth that I think we are all born with. Young children move freely secure in this knowledge, unfortunately as time goes on I think it often becomes buried by rejection, harmful messages and pain. Rediscovering this self-acceptance was key for me before I could make any lasting progress. At this point, I began making changes motivated by self-love.

My next move was to discover exercise that I loved. In the past, I'd seen exercise as a punishment for my 'failures' and so I'd workout with my insecurities acting as some kind of inner-bitch, personal trainer. I discovered dance fitness which was all about letting go and losing myself in the music. At these classes there was a whole array of body shapes moving, shimmying, shaking and giggling and I started to learn that beauty is generous, there's no one size fits all. With this shift in my mindset, I soon started losing weight and becoming more mobile. The classes were just what I needed, It's hard to be at war with your body when it's pumping adrenaline, you're making moves, flying on endorphins, and having so much fun.

Finally, I had to learn how to deal with 'failure'. This is something I struggle with, I'm a natural perfectionist and either set impossibly high standards or I'm tempted to give up. I've realised that this has been significant in how I've treated my body, I allowed myself to abuse my body because it didn't meet my standards. So I set an initial target for myself that was reachable but still quite far from what I desired. This was a huge step, to let go of what I considered to be 'ideal'. I also told myself that I wasn't going to be 'perfect' at weight loss either, I prepared myself for setbacks and accepted that unhealthy habits (mental and physical) were going to be hard to break. It was hard, we live in a society that pushes sugar at every opportunity (while telling us that the ideal body shape is slim and athletic) and we have parts of the food industry that deliberately makes products more addictive. I think it's important to acknowledge this because this environment sets us up for 'failure', it's not all 'my fault'.

Long-lasting weight loss is extremely difficult but for most people I think it can be possible. For real healthy progress, weight loss needs to be part of a bigger commitment to total mental, physical and spiritual health. My real weight loss journey hasn't really been about getting rid of fat but gaining a new understanding of myself, discovering who I really am, what I really need and then experiencing freedom.

To Round Up

It's possible that a thin person might (and this is not an exhaustive list):

- Have their life together
- Be genetically predisposed to thinness
- Work really hard at staying thin at a cost/loss to other parts of their lives
- Have a mental / eating / exercising disorder
- Have suffered trauma as a child
- Still feel fat
- Be hungry and tired
- Be unhealthy
- Die young
- None of the above

It's possible a fat person might:

- Have their life together but have had to work much harder to get there
- Be genetically pre-disposed to fatness
- Have worked really hard on their self-assurance at a cost/loss to other parts of their lives
- Be healthy
- Have suffered trauma as a child
- Have a mental / eating / exercising disorder
- Love their body
- Have rejected the natural diversity of their body, even disconnecting from it
- Live a long life
- None of the above

I really hope this section has given you pause and challenged some of the assumptions you may have around dieting and weight loss and has given you plenty of examples that fly in the face of the fantasy body. I also hope it offers reflections on fatness and out-dated links to laziness or greed or any other negative link such as, deserving of criticism or even abuse. I hope it allows you to think of fatness not as shameful or even behavioural but as a complicated weaving together of potentially many external factors, including things completely outside of our control, such as our physical differences at a biological level. I hope it gives you the opportunity to reflect that weight loss simply isn't for everyone, the way it might be for some and that that doesn't have to get in the way of healthy lifestyles or a person's value, contribution, potential or credibility. I hope to shift beliefs, just a little (actually a lot - the dial needs to move in a big way), towards putting fantasy bodies in the bin and accepting the Natural Diversity of Bodies.

How We're Making People Fat

In 2018, a feed on *Mumsnet* titled 'I hate the body positive movement' accrued 195 comments. The original poster, Raven88 explained that 'It scares me that they are leading people down a dangerous path by promoting an unhealthy lifestyle'[48]. This statement and the subsequent comments highlighted one thing… change is coming… and people are confused. You could say, the recent rise of the Body Positive Movement is a social reaction to a current norm that is glitched - the overused, exhausted use of the 'ideal body' in our cultural landscape and the harmful effects that it causes.

For the most part, most people have no idea how, the way we talk about bodies, impacts fat people or people with eating disorders for that matter. The accepted, normalised narrative around bodies - the way we believe in fantasy bodies… is making people fat. At the end of 2019, I went to a music shop to buy a soft case for my son's guitar for Christmas. Two chaps were helping me, but we had a problem. My son's electric guitar isn't symmetrical, instead on one side it has an extended 'horn'. But the cases are designed for symmetrical guitars. Between the three of us, we tried to figure out how to adapt it. Perhaps cut the lining, remove the foam, sew it up again. Nah, that'd look rubbish. Instead we decided to just sort of try and reshape or squash the foam. First the guys tried with their hands, huffing and puffing over it but it was in a complicated position. Then one said 'We need something small and heavy'. His colleague replied laughing, 'I'll go and fetch Brian[1], he's just next

[1] Names have been changed

door!' Oh how they laughed. It could play out in any workplace, in any town or city, possibly in any country in the world.

Fatness as a legitimate form of humour. No deeper consideration for *how Brian might feel*, that his colleagues have body-shamed him to a customer, a complete stranger. Or how that plays out for Brian. It pays no attention to the acute pain, shame, embarrassment, disconnection that some people feel in regard to their bodies – I wish I'd said, 'Just because it doesn't hurt you, doesn't mean it doesn't hurt him'. And can we pause for a minute and say, in no other discriminatory fashion would this be ok any more. Humour at the expense of Brian being black, or gay or disabled or any other prejudice, would not be tolerated in the way that it is still very much accepted for fat people.

My Grandma was a privileged 5'6' like I am. She used to call my Mum up and the first thing she'd ask is if she'd lost any weight. Framed her entire value on her body. Mum tells me how this used to make her head straight to the kitchen on putting the phone down. She'd fill the hole with food. In her book *Fattily Ever After*, Stephanie Yeboah tells us 'Excessive eating became my way of dealing with the bullying and the more I ate, the bigger I became which in turn lead to the increase in bullying. It was a constant circle of woe.'[49] In a brilliant put-down, James Cordon responds to Bill Maher's call for the return of fat-shaming in a viral video saying 'If making fun of fat people made them lose weight, there'd be no fat kids in schools.'[50]

Time for a tempting overgeneralisation. The best thing to do if you are overweight, is diet. Or is it? Research by Neumark-Sztianer in 2007 entitled *Why does dieting predict weight gain in adolescents?* A five-year longitudinal study. Researcher Grabe reflects on it here 'In part, dieting may lead to weight gain via the long-term adoption of behavioural patterns that are counterproductive to weight management. More specifically it shows that adolescents who reported dieting were at nearly twice the risk of being over-weight five years later *and* that those who used unhealthful weight control behaviours such as meal-skipping and diet pills, were at three times the risk.'[51]

'Research has similarly found that dieting behaviours and weight-related teasing by family members increased the risk for both disordered eating and overweight status in adolescents.' (Sanchez, et al, 2012).[52]

There is a fairly strong argument that dieting makes us fatter and I totally get how that happens. The Glitch places a false pressure, especially in the minds of young, developing people, to have the fantasy body. On appraising their naturally diverse body – which by the way, might not be unhealthy *or* overweight – while using a measure of fantasy bodies, they kick-start dieting practices. Leading to cycles of dieting and binging. Those diets don't work the way people want them to because they can't achieve the fantasy body, partly because diversity is real and natural but also because their motivation was purely for aesthetics rather than a deep personal reason, and ultimately they give up *and* eat more as a result of their deprivation or perceived failure – leading to an increased likelihood of obesity in adulthood.

I am imagining a story that goes like this, one of potentially many. A girl at around twelve or thirteen has become conscious of the fantasy world around her, perhaps she is developing quicker than other girls too. As she grows into a teenager, maybe there is a well-meaning comment or two to reinforce The Glitch. Perhaps some body-shaming among her friends, maybe even directed at her. Perhaps she puts in some serious hours going bug-eyed over social media (or for different generations reading Mizz and Just 17 or binge-watching MTV, flicking through Jackie magazine, or ogling at movie stars at the flicks). She starts to see that her body is wrong. Now this doesn't mean unhealthy, it just means that she can't identify it as being right because she can't see it anywhere in the world around her. Her body isn't valued in the world so she stops valuing it herself and decides the only thing that will help is a diet. She rejects her body. She starts a diet, begins to acknowledge 'bad' foods and food denial. Maybe she takes up more exercise, but this does actually make her *more* hungry. Perhaps being a teenager is tough and she would love to turn to the 'forbidden' food for comfort. Also teenagers are madly growing and developing so hunger is natural. Maybe in a fit of frustration and vulnerability, which she might not be able to put her finger on, she breaks her vow and binge eats all the forbidden fruits she has felt denied of. And perhaps she is half a pound heavier the next time she hits the scales. And so, the cycle repeats. The weight actually creeps up and one day the doctor confirms that she has slipped into the obese category. Perhaps she doesn't appreciate being told what to do with her own body. Perhaps the efforts she makes don't give the desired (fantasy body) results quick enough, so what is the point? No this doesn't kick-start any better attempts at weight loss and it isn't until she has a meaningful personal reason to do something about it, that anything really changes.

The Don't Tell Me What To Do Rule

Remember back in the last chapter, when I talked about us all having different interests. I've never played football – that's not true – I have played it once, not a fan. I've seen it on the telly but it has never sparked the remotest interest in me beyond the patriotic. And yet, it's popular, four billion fans think so, there must be something in it! Probably, if I gave it enough of my attention, I could get engaged and work out how they manage to fill so many TV hours talking about it, I could even become passionate about it. I just haven't been brought up with it, I don't truly understand it, have never really taken the time to, and my life is full of other interests so it's fine.

I'm now imagining how I'd feel if someone told me I *had* to enjoy football. Whaaaaat! Hell no, *you* enjoy it! It's now gone from something I *might* want to explore on my own, to something I *definitely* don't want to do. I don't get anything out of it. I'm not doing that! I wonder if that's every fat person who's been recommended to diet and exercise ever? When we tell people what they 'have' to or even 'ought' to or repeated enough times what they 'could' do, it robs them of their self-agency. Let's stop doing that.

The Exercise vs Humiliation Rule

However for some, it's not just a case of 'I'm just not that in to exercise'. Instead, it's rooted in self-preservation. The Glitch means that for some fat people and especially very fat people, exercise is off the table. Through my work (which we'll come to), I've had *so* many people report that the abuse they have experienced while exercising, either outdoors but more readily, in a gym (oh *those* places - the inclusive ones, full of diverse imagery! Not!) has made the experience too painful to endure. Think about it, even one painful, shaming comment, would be enough to make me hyper-aware of my body as a target. By the way, a huge percentage, (almost all) of the men I've interviewed about this, told me their body shame / dissatisfaction started for them in the changing rooms at school.

Postscript from one of my first readers: Another example of the problem with gyms – the standard size towels they hand out. If you are 'gym' sized you can wrap up as you enter/exit the showers – any bigger and it just becomes a glorified hand towel and you are left with the dilemma of which body part to cover up, knowing it will just draw attention to the rest. I end up giving up and just strutting through the changing rooms naked but that's clearly not for everyone!

And Another Thing

I want to touch on another aspect of exercise, the exercise as punishment rule. Exercise isn't always therapeutic, sometimes people are using it as punishment or as part of the complex routine tied up in their eating disorder. Exercise addiction being another part of the illness that doesn't get enough airtime.

The Restriction / Rebellion Rule

I remember from my own experience of restriction and rebellion, just how strong that pull was to stop stopping. I wanted to eat no sugar but I also wanted really badly to stop not eating sugar and always wondered when the break would come, what the trigger would be and then… *free flow that sugar into me.* Aubrey Gordon talks about this dynamic causing her to 'fetishise' food[53]. Depriving myself only made me super alert to what I was missing. Because in all of the commentary and content around dieting, weight loss, health and longevity we fail to acknowledge one really important factor. Food is fun! Food is delicious. Food is joy, community, relaxation, tradition, essential, nutritious… I love food! As soon as we ban a food, we also create a dynamic of mental toil, inner conflict, punishment or failure. It's *so* healthy, honestly!

The Depression Cycle

You can see how the points from this chapter already would predispose someone to depression. In fact, the links from depression, shame, sadness, anxiety and self-criticism to obesity are well documented: 'We found bidirectional associations between depression and obesity: obese persons had a 55% increased risk of developing depression over time, whereas depressed persons had a 58% increased risk of becoming obese.'[54]

I don't blame you if reading this you think, this all feels culturally so messed up, complicated and entrenched, how will it ever change? What's the point in trying? I know… I sometimes feel that way too. It feels too big. However as we'll see, it's not about the culture changing, it's just about you, me and us. So let's crack on…

The Angel and the Devil Paradox

Tell me something. A person comes to you, tells you how valued you are, how much they appreciate your work and effort, they want you to know you belong and are valued. Because of this, your talents would be really helpful in solving a problem they have. Would you mind?

Another person comes to you. They moan about the weather, they moan about the traffic, they tell you that you're rubbish too. Can't you just hurry up? Don't you want to try harder? Be better? Not sure this place is for you mate. Oh, by the way, can you help them, with this problem they have? How easy would you find it to help them?

This second person describes the atmosphere, the landscape, the norm, that many fat people live with, in the world but often internalised in their heads too. Being ridiculed – still legitimately! Being harassed, embarrassed, abused, verbally, emotionally, physically, being excluded, invisible. It can present itself in seemingly innocuous comments, reinforcing fantasy bodies, such as a throwaway comment about a fat Labrador, or a well-meaning suggestion for a diet, recommendation of a surgeon, even a comment that they've lost weight, it all reinforces The Glitch and skews their footing against them. This can show itself in some people being apparently incapable to not mention difference or stare at it, like toddlers. Or some people offering their unsolicited, knowing advice for marginalised people with no actual knowledge of their experience. It can be a fat person having to reassure thinner friends that *they're* not fat. Having to hear fantasy body coding, even if not directed at them. All of this is *not* helping fat people become thinner. It's all more noise that gets in the way of that person and their own personal journey to health or connection to their own body. It doesn't help fat people help themselves if they want it. It interrupts it, even if it's just you saying *you* need to lose weight, it reminds them, you think they're not good enough and they too have to change, even if you don't think that. You can easily show yourself up to be fairly narrow in your world-view and experiences.

Equally the devil might also be in their head, creating yet another barrier to health. So how easy would it be to help yourself in that situation? I for one would find making healthy progress, should I want to, in a cultural atmosphere of acceptance and support, much easier. Which brings me on to...

Inclusion and How to Become and Ally

(Friend, partner, mother, father, sister, brother, daughter, colleague, boss, fellow bus-rider, whatever.)

You know, it isn't possible to hold and centre the needs, concerns, unique viewpoints and experiences, esoteric to every possible marginalisation. All at once. All the time. We'd never function. It's not possible to filter every comment that comes out of our mouth. God I've said some dumb stuff in my time. You might be reading this and feeling *gasp* *I've done that, I've said that.* It's normal. Don't fret. That said there is a strong argument for better homelife, social, cultural, workplace, academic and medical inclusion. Actually not just to include everyone and give a step up to those who are experiencing marginalisation in life, as ethically highbrow as that would be, but also to help take The Glitch apart, piece by piece - for everyone, including us, our loved ones, our future generations. Because The Glitch isn't getting any better. Hell no. It's getting steadily worse.

Can I start by saying, 'inclusion', buzz-word that it is, is not the gold standard. Inclusion is the very least we can do. Inclusion is our clunky route from here to an equal world - where inclusion isn't even a consideration. Now that would be the gold standard. But for now *sigh* we will have to work with the concept of inclusion and the idea that the world and all its bounty is for everyone. Hopefully by this point in the book, I will have given plenty of reasons to support this and include body shape and size under that broad umbrella term. I hope I've sufficiently demonstrated that most fat people don't choose to be that way and that body shape is largely out of our control. This impacts the inclusion conversation because I believe a bias towards believing people could and should control their bodies is what currently keeps body shape / image out of most inclusion conversations. Indeed many organisations and initiatives designed for inclusivity, still find it hard to put a fat person on their marketing materials as the visual of inclusion. But if inclusion isn't about including everyone, then – beyond the 'optics'. If inclusion isn't inclusive, then what is the point?

Oh, didn't I say? Because currently it isn't. The equality conversation doesn't currently embrace body difference, body variations, there's a good chance that your workplace's Equality Statement doesn't mention it and it's because we are sadly lacking learning and knowledge in this area beyond a narrow narrative. You head over to your nearest Equality Policy, you most likely won't find it there. Under The Equalities Act? Nope. Theses are prejudices not upheld by these otherwise protecting mechanisms. Not a protected discrimination in this modern twenty-first-century world. Anti-fatness, or fatphobia is still fair game. Indeed:

In analysing results from its famed implicit bias tests, Harvard University Lead Researcher, Carey Goldberg reports: 'Contrary to the assumption that implicit (conscious) attitudes don't change, we found that actually, three out of the six implicit attitudes have shown change. Sexuality attitudes, at an implicit level, have changed by about 33 percent over the past decade, whereas race and skin-tone perceptions also changed, just at a slower rate: about 17 percent for race attitudes and 15 percent for skin tone attitude.

Age, disability and body weight attitudes haven't changed; actually, body weight attitudes even showed a slight tendency that they're becoming worse over time.'[55]

I can't speak for fat people. What I do know is that the loss to my life, through issues around self-esteem and body image, because of The Glitch are merely the tip of the iceberg in contrast to those who live in fat and marginalised bodies. In fact for those people, it isn't a 'Glitch'. It's often abuse, trauma and can be severely life-limiting – unnecessary loss doesn't quite cover it. And many have put up with it their whole lives.

To truly understand and invoke empathy for what that feels like, we can educate ourselves. Reading around this subject would give us a much better grasp of the daily toil experienced by those living in fat or marginalised bodies. This might require you first to put down any pre-conceived notions about the fantasy body and pay attention. Again, read Aubrey's book, and Stephanie Yeboah's *Fattily Ever After* to gain some insight and context of their worlds.

Next you can check your feeds. Are you living in an echo chamber that reflects a fantasy world back to you? That leaves you unchallenged to see things differently? The trend of creating a social media feed – especially on Instagram - which is just reams and reams and reams of the person's body, has become totally normalised. As has using filters. My daughter sent me a gif the other day of her face on the White Queen in the film *Alice in Wonderland*, further stretching the lengths we can go to, to leave reality for dust. We have created a society where it has become a norm and readily accepted, especially in younger girls/women, to post repeated images of yourself on social media. The Galleries of Selfies! They often come with associated complimentary comments from friends. Where are the rest of their lives? Where are the books they read, the causes they champion, the passions they love, the people they admire, the shows they watch, the craft they create? I mean I get it, if you took away bodies from the traditional format of magazines, there'd be next to nothing left. Yet as content creators - all of us -

I do wonder at the motivation of folks who relentlessly share just images of themselves. Either they're selling me their body – the image or idea of it obvs not their actual body! Or they have a real need for reassurance and might be a bit in need of help. Not sure truly healthy people endlessly share pics of themselves without motivation (such as being a model, bopo activist or like I said, to sell a concept – their personal training business for example). I'd argue there's still room even on these feeds for other interests / opinion. A bit of balance. I'm wondering if it's a form of anxiety? Do they serve to reassure? To validate? I'm sure not much thought goes in to the why, but in doing this, we've got to ask, is it healthy? (I can sense such eyerolls coming my way right now). But even posts, shared under the hashtag of #bodypositivity are a reminder to think again about our bodies. This version of The Glitch serves to once again, value the appearance of our bodies above everything else.

The links between viewing or uploading selfies and lower body satisfaction are already well documented. Talking about this, one BBC article, urges us to 'Put down your phone' before immediately also urging us to 'Join 900,000+ Future fans (what's a 'Future fan'?) by liking us on Facebook, or follow us on Twitter or Instagram.'[56] Oh heck, now I've found another glitch! Anyone waking up from a twenty-year coma and being introduced to social media, would be hard pressed to understand what happened to people having hobbies, interests, talents, opinions relating to anything other than bodies.

Do your feeds reflect the natural diversity of bodies? They could and that content is a great source of learning for us all. It's bitesize and regular input into our heavily conditioned brains. Follow the hashtags: #realbodies #effyourbeautystandards #fatliberation #inclusionrevolution #fatactivism #bigblackandbeautiful #transpride #gaypride #lovemychub #disabilityempowerment

#plussizemen #nosizefitsall #nonairbrushed #bodyconfidence #thisgirlcan or anything else that *isn't* to do with bodies! Oh there are so many that could open up your world and once you start you can find yourself down a magical rabbit hole of diversity and reality. There's still some fantasy pics in there too just scroll, scroll, scroll. I'd also like to propose #DitchTheGlitch #realbodies and #naturaldiversity to gain traction. Another tool in this activity… 'unfollow'. You are in charge of your feed, it's your life. Make it exactly what you want. Follow what interests you, what lights you up, what you care about and ditch the endless bodies.

Another form of allyship is simply ~~talking~~ listening to people. Not every marginalised person will want to talk to you about what can be a really painful subject. Some may be wary, however, if they do, reach out, don't argue, justify, or talk over their lived experience. Just listen. Here's what happened when I ventured into a conversation with one of my contacts:

Body Stories
Nick Butcher

Nick (laughing): … the only nice thing that has come out of 2020 is I don't see many people during lockdown for them to comment on my height!

Emi (laughing): That's not a good thing! Tell me how tall you are.
Nick: So I am 6'7' I got to about sixteen years old and stopped measuring. At the time I was so annoyed by it!

Emi: What was it like at school?

Nick: School was tough insofar as, any difference that people can pick up on, they do, I was always the tallest kid in the school, from literally being five years old. I was also very thin, so it stood out that I was quite tall. Going into secondary school, it impacted me more. Until then I was taller than the other kids but not taller than the teachers. I would say I was the tallest in the school. You know, kids are kids and what stands out was the name calling. I did let it get to me, probably not outwardly but it did, otherwise I wouldn't be talking about it now, twenty years later!

In my mid-twenties I got a really good group of friends - everyone had a nick name. One guy came up with the name 'Tall Boy' and it stuck. I know they meant no harm but every time it was said, it was like a knife being jabbed into my chest. I'd just have to smile and be like 'Yeah great…'

They're not malicious people and I'll happily admit that I'd call others nicknames, but it would just get my back up when anyone mentioned it. They just didn't realise that it was horrible to be reminded of your size! Occasionally, now, I might see one of them and they'll go 'Alright Tall Boy' and I'll be like eugh (rolls eyes). Don't do it! They don't realise they're saying it, if they heard me say this, they'd be so apologetic. It brings in everything from year dot.
I like being tall and I like that I'm memorable, hopefully for more than just my height, it does give me an emphasis in a room but I'm also aware that I'm larger than life, so when you go and give someone a hug, you realise that you're quite an imposing person, so you retreat as well, you don't want to be that big, sort of lurchy person.

Emi: Overwhelming?

Nick: Yeah exactly. When someone comes up and asks about your height or when you're in the queue in Sainsbury's and people are openly talking behind your back about how tall you are, it's incredible I've had people measure themselves up to me, thinking I wouldn't notice. I don't want to say anything because, I never want to come across as aggressive as that can change into conflict quickly, so you just have to take it. I'll be honest with you, you feel like the smallest person in the room and you're very aware that you stand out. I also had people throw stuff at me at concerts and say 'Can you get out of the way?' I wouldn't mind if I was at the front, I but I'm usually stood by the sound desk at the back.

Emi: All of this doesn't really describe your character.

Nick: Absolutely, it's hard when you're young and you're trying to establish your identity, I remember being at a party once and everyone was talking about the qualities they liked in the other people in the room 'Such and such is funny and intelligent, such and such is good at music etc' and they come to me and they went 'Well you're tall' even though I know I'm plenty of other things!

You can guarantee every day someone will say, 'How tall are you?', 'How's the weather up there?', 'Do you play basketball?' and you can just recycle these questions. I don't mind talking about it if they're genuinely lovely and interested. Some people say it I think because of their own insecurities and almost wish they had a bit of my height and feel that I've won some sort of lottery and they didn't get that, and they can be nasty.

Emi: Do you have any examples?

Nick: When I was going out a lot more when I was younger, afterwards in the kebab shop, I've had people pick fights with me literally because they're the little guy and they want to beat up the tall guy, you just don't want to be involved with it. So that's not nice.

When I went into the world of work, I was in the car industry at the time. I'd be meeting the general public, going up to customers, I'd be trying to do my job talking through this car and the person would go 'I'm really sorry, how tall are you?' I can't tell you how small that makes you feel. They seem to think that because I'm tall, and I should be proud of that, which I am, they can say what they like to me. If I go back with a bit of a sarcastic comment, it's my problem but if someone came up to you and said 'You're fat' or 'short', you'd be offended.

Emi: Of course you would.

Nick: I can always tell the quality of someone if they mention my height or not. The people I get on with the best are the people who have never really mentioned my height. They just see me for me. The people that really annoy me bring it up straight away and you can tell the people who are being nasty or not, trying a bit of one-up-man-ship by the way they say it and usually they won't let it go. With others they may just think they're making conversation. I've been in very rare situations where I've met someone taller than me. I've been like 'Wow!' and you think, *Oh God, what am I doing*? But I've never gone up and asked them how tall they are! In fact, when meeting people my height you end up having this same conversation, you empathise with each other.

Emi: The funny thing about us is, we've never actually met (I contacted Nick after hearing him on the *See Within Podcast*, he is an HR specialist - it was nothing to do with bodies, which just goes to reinforce how, so many of us are impacted by negative body image.) and I can't tell that you're really tall, in fact I'm quite surprised, because I can only see your head! (It's 2020 and everything is on Zoom) But I will say that if I'd just met you, I could have blundered into saying something like that, purely out of surprise, almost like 'Oh, wow! You are tall!' sort of a comment.

Nick: And I don't blame people for that.

Emi: I think what I would not know, before having this conversation, is just how frustrating it must be, for it to be constant, it must be so boring, like a part of your life, that you have to do that extra bit of work that other people don't.

Nick: Either someone's asking it or they're about to. I have to say if I meet someone who is really small, they're less likely to talk about it. They know the rubbish they get for being really small, they'll know what I'm getting for being tall. It's more your average person who can't seem to accept the fact that I'm taller than them. For some reason it completely defines their thoughts on me.

Emi: I guess, there are no days when you get to be inconspicuous. You must feel very exposed.

Nick: When I left school I didn't leave with much and I was going for an interview. I'd just left my first job in the car industry I was keen on staying in the industry so went for an interview in a dealership in Weybridge and the guy who interviewed me, he was a really nice guy, I felt the conversation went really well, you know, I answered the right questions and I was a competent sales person but at the interview, he said something along the lines of 'Yeah, it's all good, there's just one concern that I've got.' He said, 'Will you stand up for me?' so I stood up feeling like a piece of meat. And he just looked at me and said 'I just think you're too tall. You'd be too imposing for the customers.' So all the insecurities I had came back, I thought, *Oh my God, it's in the world of work, it's going to hold back my career!* I left there thinking that was my problem, because I was eighteen years old. If it happened now, I'd tell the bloke where to go, but that's at 36 years-of-age. That's one tiny example in my life.

Emi: So how did you move forward from that and get more confidence?

Nick: I was lucky that shortly afterwards I went to work for a dealership with a great owner who said 'Right Nick, you're coming to work for me, I'm going to show you this business' and my height didn't matter. It wasn't until then that I got a bit of confidence. I went into the job as one person, three years later I came out such a different person, a boy-to-man experience. The odd customer would mention it but ultimately, I was there because I was good at my job. So for me it was my mid-twenties where I had a different mind-set because I started to achieve things. And sometimes my height was to my advantage because I'd walk into a room and people would remember me. You know if you back that up with being a decent human being as well… Now if I go into a room, I use everything I've got to try and be that little 1% better than the next person and if it makes me more memorable, as long as people aren't nasty about that, I'm OK with that. In the great scheme of things, it's their problem not mine. I'm pretty content with who I am and what I do but it's just been very eye-opening.

Emi: It must be so frustrating. I just hope, well, people may think before they speak.

Nick: Yeah, it's one of these things where it's time for me to talk about it, it's the sixteen, seventeen, eighteen-year-olds who aren't ok with it. I'm not going to lie and say it goes away but it's the understanding that it's the other person's problem not mine and it's something I should be proud about.

Nick Butcher runs Ignition Human Performance – Leadership and Performance lessons from F1 and motorsport to help unlock people performance in business.

Being and Ally Continued…

To be an ally, we can take a lesson from Nick, and try and think before we speak. But we can also speak up. When you or someone nearby is on the receiving end of prejudice, we can call them out with: 'Did you mean for that to sound so offensive?' Or similar.

We can also be mindful to focus on those who fall under the category of having a marginalised body and by extension living a marginalised life. We can step our privilege aside and give *them* a platform to be heard, on whatever stage we play on.

The Wood and the Trees

It's not always easy to reach the people on the blunt end of inequality, those least affected by it. I was thinking this the other day while I was walking in Delamere Forest and I think the forest is a good analogy.

At the edge of the forest, where the wind hits, the trees were growing at a stoop, buffeting the elements, taking the strain of the real or external world. Our marginalised people live like this, cast out, different, with more work to do. They've made their growth under harsher conditions and grown anyway. Buffeted against everyday comments that may, or may not, be barbed.

As you walk further in, this happens less and less until right in the middle, trees are standing straight and true. And they have no idea, the hardships of the trees on the outer edges. And as they don't even know about the hardships, how could they help? So many privileged people, like the internal trees, lack understanding, knowledge or experience and stay uninformed or turn away from the problem. Maybe it's even easier to believe in fantasy lives in that space. Our major hurdle then, is to find ways to engage those people with the sharp end of inequality, no matter how uncomfortable, inconvenient or costly.

Listen we live in an achievement-driven world – making mistakes, being wrong, failures have been demonised rather than celebrated as a means to growth (can we have a re-brand over here please) so it's not always that easy to take, to acknowledge. Regardless, it is for those people who are blinkered to find empowering ways to accept and absorb the information. All too often I see people faced with addressing inequality or their own blundering boob and either declining to comment or taking it personally. We need to find classier, more accepted, less defensive ways to have our awareness raised. A kind of new breed of 'my bad'. I want to say, I'm especially thinking of white men here but it's not exclusively them, who could stand to learn there's something very sexy about awareness. It is in those people recognising the position they hold and then listening. It is in us recognising our position there, if we fill one, and using our privilege to do something. Building protection around the boundary of the forest. Aside from anything else, I fear we may rather swiftly become extinct, out of touch, if we resist. The future is coming, and it's much more tolerant and diverse. Hold on to your hats if you're not ready!

And remember inclusion and allyship isn't yet about everyone being equal, it needs to be about giving a step up to those who need it most. But it is *for* everyone, we all would benefit from breaking The Glitch and fostering a more inclusive society. By getting out of our echo chambers, learning what solutions other people have to problems, by truly revealing individuals' value once we see past our bias, benefitting from it and re-connecting with reality and our own bodies. For it to work the *most* effectively, it would require everyone to get on board.

Your Body Connection

Building Back the Bond

'A woman obsessed with the reduction of her flesh may be revealing the fact that she is alienated from a natural source of female power and has not been allowed to develop a reverential feeling for her body.'

Kim Chernin

Kim Chernin was a psychotherapist and one of the first academics to really focus on body image, eating disorders and women. Her 1981 book, The Obsession, Reflections on the Tyranny of Slenderness[57] became a best-seller. Remember her because we're going to come back to her in a future chapter.

As far back as 1947, philosopher, Simone de Beauvoir noted something similar. That we are too quick to identify with a 'spirit of seriousness', 'certain abstractions at the expense of individual freedom' that in the pursuit of perfection 'countless individuals' are sacrificed. She was in support of a code of ethics that 'values the freedom of each individual'.

'Human beings enmeshed in their own unique situations and engaged in their own projects.' [58]

Simone de Beauvoir

So we need to start asking questions of ourselves. We can start with, who am I? And what do I want? Sorry maybe I should have said, this section is going to be about getting honest and being open with ourselves. As Chenin notes, 'Many women would rather work towards the body our culture admires than analyse the reasons they dislike their body as it is.' Go gently with this, ok. It might be worth working with a pen and a notebook.

So where is your personal power? Hint, it's not in a screen. What do we mean by power? Well, you are already working with your personal power, it's how any of us get anything done! But we might not be using all of it. Or even most of it.

To recap, believing in fantasy bodies is: wasting our attention, money, energy, our lives. It is suffocating. Every negative thought, misguided comment, mental food or exercise transaction, assigning our core value to false things, is all a waste and it creates unnecessary stress in our bodies and a disconnection from ourselves.

Your personal power deficit might look like: all of that energy that you put into the rightness of your body; all of that attention that isn't focussing on things that light you up, but instead on fitting into a version of ourselves that doesn't exist; or a lifetime's effort to prove your worth, when there was never anything wrong with you to begin with.

Personal power can connect you to self-acceptance, self-apology and self-forgiveness, turning cogs to unstick yourself and grease the wheels of moving on. It can help you ask for what you want and feeling deserving of it. Progress. What could we do with that power? What would you like to do with it? There is a lot to care about, to heal this world, small – in our homes and big – on our planet. What is our purpose if it doesn't lie in the way our bodies look?

What's more, when we measure our worth instead by how loved we are and how we love, by how useful, valuable, talented we are, what we contribute, how we can help, progress, what is in our capacity to achieve. When we tap into our unique selves, to the things that make us, us. To the things that give our lives meaning, that remind us why we're here. When we assess our worth based on the people we choose to share our lives with and those that find their way to us, on how much we laugh, hug, thank, create, taste, hear… then it starts getting real, achievable, within grasp, progressive, joyful, happy, successful and Goddammit it's powerful!

To do that and show up as our most effective, authentic, undistracted selves for our worlds, we need to fit our oxygen masks first, and next we need to visit one really important and sometimes troublesome question.

Do I like myself?

Do we like ourselves enough to start caring about ourselves in a deeper, primal way. It's important to note, that question can bring up some pretty strong emotions (and sometimes resistance – jot down anything that comes up). The Glitch isn't packaged for us to like ourselves. Also cultural norms and habits have formed around putting ourselves down, self-deprecation, not 'showing off'. Other people's agendas might have kept us small, apologetic. We may even have had some early programming, or on-going input from our loved ones about how we're not good enough. If that's the case, please, please, please talk this through in a safe space, be it with a partner, a friend, a therapist. The Hub of Hope app connects you with services close to you which can help. Full details at the back of the book.

I want you to visualise your power, you choose the colour, the form, the shape. Does it live in your body, or outside of it? Now imagine you're in a stadium, surrounded by everyone else's power too. Feels electric, that buzz, but that's not even close to the potential power we wield if we ALL could just tap into our freedom, our creativity, our passions, intentions, our self-belief. Our power can be amplified or our power can be dimmed. The Glitch, along with other things, dims it. So let's get to work. First, some practical things to consider – you don't have to but you could:

Ditch your scales. You will know if you put on weight or if you lose it, you don't need a daily commentary and emotional fall-out on that.

Ditch the number or type of mirrors in your home. Do you really need them too?

Ditch clothes that haven't fit you for ages or that only fitted you fleetingly. And don't buy more, to diet into. Bin that pressure.

Ditch 'wish weights' and acknowledge them when they float into your mind.

Do journal all the yuck that might come up in this process. Getting it out, onto the page can be a real release but it can also make it easier to appraise it objectively and spot logic flaws.

Do write your body a love letter

Do conserve your personal power by ditching The Glitch and getting real

Do encourage your friends to do so too, or spend time with people already on this path.

So, let's do this and then from a place of wholeness, go after whatever it is you want life to offer you - your purpose - stronger, healthier and more rooted in reality. The most common objection I get to doing this work is 'I don't have the time', which I inner chuckle at, because here's a chance to free up your time and so much more. However, like I've mentioned, you can't know what you don't know; you also can't unknow what you now know. You're already changing and thinking differently with a load of new perspectives now whirring away inside you. It's what you choose to do with it next that counts. That bit is all up to you, are you ready to do the inner work?

Hopefully by this point we have plenty of motivation to Stop Believing in Fantasy Bodies and just Ditch The Glitch. But how are we actually going to do it? First we are going to deeply internalise our new mantra:

I don't believe in fantasy bodies
I don't believe in fantasy bodies
I don't believe in fantasy bodies
I don't believe in fantasy bodies

And we repeat it any time we're faced with… a fantasy body or glitchy reasoning or uninformed comments. So there's that. Now I want to take you back to where I can pinpoint what shifted in me to start connecting myself back to my body. Are you sitting comfortably?

What Cancer Taught Me

I found this blog from Autumn 2016, I wrote it before I saw the *Embrace* film, before M&S and my 'Realise you are enough, exactly as you are' line. Before I realised this would be the foundation of my work…

'In a gentle way, you can shake the world'

Gandhi

I began to write this blog (Mummy One Boob) four years ago (2012) when I was diagnosed, because I knew I'd learn my big lessons through this journey. I wanted to show others what those lessons were, without them having to go through the hard times. I read, I watched, I thought... At times it has been a baffling, conflicted journey. One that raised more questions than it answered. But then I learnt a lesson. A lesson to put those questions to bed. I realised that the lesson I learnt has a much wider-reaching impact. I'm going to be bold here and claim it has the potential to heal us, our world and create compassion in places we least expect.

Now for the exciting stuff! This lesson can also take:

- the heat out of arguments
- the juice out of gossip
- the failure out of trying
- the hate out of self-hating

Imagine a world where all of those things are replaced by something better!

Helping us to:

- love our closest more
- thrive in our relationships
- find gratitude for all we have
- achieve satisfaction
- adore ourselves and be OK with that
- stop giving up
- realise our dreams

It's a short lesson, in fact it comes down to just one word. One word, if we could neutralise it or even remove it and its meaning from our vocabulary, it would revolutionise our lives. Just shining a light on it can create a tangible shift in perception. It did for me, anyway.

Do you know what it is?

Maybe you already do.

What this word reflects is a social dis-ease, one that we don't appreciate is constricting us. A bit like the Emperor's New Clothes, we live to its standards, accept them, hurt ourselves with them. Even when we know deep down it's all complete codswobble. When you know the word, you'll be like 'Of course!' but you don't live that way. None of us do and it's about time we changed.

We didn't create this 'norm' and we CAN change. Speaking

personally, learning this message and using it regularly, has revolutionised my life. It has helped me find more happy. I mostly wasn't, now I mostly am. That word…?

Perfect!

So simple right? So let's recap. This message will take:

- the heat out of arguments – you're not perfect and neither am I
- the juice out of gossip – she/he's not perfect
- the failure out of trying – I'm not perfect
- the hate out of self-hating – oh yeah, I'm not perfect

In fact, practicing imperfection has brought me relief and comfort from life's frustrations big and small. It has genuinely helped me to...

- love my closest more
- thrive in my relationships
- help me find gratitude for all I have
- feel more satisfied with my life
- appreciate myself
- stop giving up
- realise my dreams
- accept my health
- even face my own death

If I didn't need to be perfect, I could accept all the parts of me that I don't like. I've tried to achieve happiness through perfection thinking – maybe you recognise it – if I could just have the perfect: house, body, job, holiday, man, woman, kids, parents, siblings, friends… everything would be rosy. Often our thinking isn't as simple as that. It can be a part of our programming that is buried deeper inside, but I know for many of us, it is there. As Elizabeth Kesses notes:

'We are at breaking point with our obsession with perfection'[59]

What I've found in fact is I only find happiness with a deep acceptance of myself and others - when I practice being imperfect. And I have practiced it a lot! And I have got it wrong... a lot! Learnt it, forgotten it, remembered it. Rinse and repeat because we're not programmed this way, it's easier to revert to type.

It's when I attach success – at work, home, in relationships - to perfection, it causes further problems. When only a perfect outcome will do, it clouds my ability to feel satisfaction, fulfilment and that buzzword - gratitude. And don't get me wrong, I know, it's hard to let go of what you thought was real. It takes practice. It doesn't happen overnight. For many of us as kids with conscientious parents, our formative behaviour was sized up against perfection. This behaviour is good, this behaviour is bad; in order for us to learn, there were rarely exceptions. I'm a parent and I get why it had to be that way. So there's an unlearning to do.

We've been conditioned in these ideas – as we grew older, the media got involved. If an advertiser can, however subtly or blatantly, find a chink in our armour, then ca-ching! We're sold; they're rich. Because we see the ideal, we like the ideal, we buy into the ideal. The ideal even feels safe in an unpredictable world. We momentarily (or longer) forget, the ideal isn't real darling…

It has become such a natural and accepted way of life, we don't even recognise it as a message being pumped into our brains. Think of how we manage our online presence, that that is even a thing. We've become pro's in styling, editing, staging, primping, selfies… what are we trying to achieve… You see that chink… it's you. It's us. It's the keystone of our imperfect, beautiful, challenging, wonderful, magnificent world. When you come at life assuming its imperfections, it's a miracle that we pull anything off at all! This makes it easier be grateful for triumphs big and small.

So my approach isn't about 'self improvement', there's no need. It's about self-actualising, self-noticing, about self-forgiving, self-compassion, and seeing just what that can do for you and your life. We're not working towards a goal here, there doesn't need to be a goal, you're not perfect, I'm sorry chicken, you never will be. But you can have more happy and start today.

What isn't perfect, about you, about your life? Notice how you feel about that. Don't throw mental stones at it. Don't brush it under the carpet. It takes some guts to just look at it. That feeling is trying to tell you something, it's up to you to listen and from there real growth can happen. If you like you can learn a prompt or two to get you through. Here's one that brings me regular relief...

It's OK that I'm not all… right.

Notice where we're being sold perfect and the good things that are imperfect. We can reinforce it with…

'Ah that's not perfect… cool!'

'Loving the honesty'

"That imperfect thing, it's totally natural poppet'

'I appreciate that real <whatever>'

And if you're feeling really righteous…

'I'm not buying into that perfection deception'

These days I would say: I don't believe in fantasy <whatever – bodies, relationships, homes, holidays…>

What all this doesn't mean is don't try. Do try; aim high. Excel! Try things you don't think will work. Think big. And when days are hard and things go wrong, congratulate yourself, you're human! 0% robot. I know this can be the starting point of a beautiful journey where people can: find their great love; create a healthy atmosphere in their body; save money; make money; heal connections; reach goals; feel good… I've travelled it myself. But it needs to shift into a social movement – like recycling, or… seatbelt wearing. We must demand it of ourselves and the world and we are starting to. It's nice to see.

'We can't direct the wind, but we can adjust the sails'[60]

Thomas S. Monson.

How we feel is up to us and it can be learnt. I've been to the edge and survived. This is what I was meant to learn. So let's re-wire some of that programming, restore the reality balance and connect ourselves back together. Time, I think for a…

Tempting Overgeneralisation

Thin people have good relationships with their bodies. Not true, many thin people have messed up relationships with their bodies and aren't as happy as you might think. People who have good relationships with their bodies are not necessarily thin or have a close version of the ideal body image. People who have a good relationship with their bodies have either been given good messaging about bodies from birth, through an enlightened teacher / parent / carer, or they've been forced to put in the work in the form of deep personal motivation.

Through my work as a body therapist, I have found it to be true, that people who have suffered physical trauma are often those people who have a healthy body relationship based on real values. It is as though their bodies have given them permission to accept them, in the knowledge they can never go back. Like me, their hopes of achieving an ideal body are gone, so let's see what's left. They may be incentivised to make peace with their bodies, often through drastic changes to their body. And actually, it's a bit of a hoax, a mind bender. Actually, everyone has the capacity to make peace with their bodies… the problem is not everyone can be bothered, will make time, even though The Glitch will rob us of more in the long run, not everyone feels they have the permission (near death often gives that) and not everyone knows how.

And that is a barrier to good health and must account for so much wasted opportunity to feel good, enjoy life, live in the moment. The 'I'll be happy when I've lost x weight' phenomenon. Enjoyable life is happening now – don't miss it! I want to show how this can manifest for us with a body story from my best friend, wing woman and fellow trauma survivor.

Body Stories
Leana Hughes

When I was 22, I was involved in a motorcycle accident. As a result, I lost four and a half inches of my tibia. It is a miracle I still have a left leg. Thanks to the fall of the Berlin wall, Russian bone-saving ingenuity made its way to our shores. Techniques used on horses during the war is what saved my leg. Thank you, Mr Illizarov with your bone-stretching cleverness!

As you can imagine, this was a lengthy and painful process, taking over a year to accomplish bone-to-bone docking. Try to imagine what a leg looks like minus a tibia and half a fibula. It looked like a shark had a nice chomp from my leg. With muscle taken from my calf, and skin harvested from my thigh, I became a patch work doll. I used to have a birthmark on the piece of skin they removed to cover up my shin bone. I remember still being a bit disappointed that my birthmark had now become a smudge. Like a mosquito on a windshield!

The year I spent in and out of hospital generated a strange connection / disconnection with my body. It was all we ever talked about. Licking my emotional wounds and changing my dressings was my daily routine. I'd say this part was my CONNECTION with my body, but it was certainly not an appreciation or a love for it. As can be expected, my body image was in tatters if you judge from how my leg looked and how people stared at the oversized external fixator frame I was lobbing around with me. But here comes the unhealthy, but looking at the bright side, wonky thinking – at least yanking a big metal cage around helped me keep the weight off! Not forgetting the energy it takes for a body to repair itself. This is where the DISCONNECT is evident – I felt pleased that at least I was skinny. Maybe people would rather now look at my weight, rather than my leg. Obviously, I was traumatised and it's very clear when I look back at photos, how frail I was. Still, I have vivid memories of staring in the mirror, feeling very satisfied and obviously not looking down at the ghastly sight that was the leg.

Almost 20 years on… It's funny, you'd think I'd be OK with my extra rolls and wobbles I collected over the years, considering I came to accept the appearance of my leg, but I hadn't. I have no problem showing my scars anymore, but you wouldn't catch me dead in a bikini! A mangled leg now almost feels socially acceptable over 40 something blubber in a cossie. The width of my thighs and the way my belly concertinas when I sit, this feels shameful. It's funny how I managed to fine-tune this external evaluation. To suit me. To suit how I believe people will judge. Scars = poor you. You're so brave. Fat = gross. You're so weak. Gosh, can we be any more cruel to ourselves? I know my body image ideals come from childhood. Years of reading Cosmo, hearing how Mum is on another diet, watching music videos. From going to modelling school to admiring the bikini clad girls in cigarette ads (that's how mature I am!).

My views have taken a turn in the last two years. It might be wisdom, it might be talks with my best friend. It might be self-acceptance, self-love and the ability to not give a fuck anymore. I've grown up. I've started to see past the rolls and wobbles. I started to look at my leg and invited it to show me what it can do. To not go by the narrative with I am less-abled, but to trust my body and to see what I've got. I exercise a lot, although only to the capacity my leg and back can last, but I DO IT. And when I can't anymore, I rest (and take my painkillers). But I don't do it any more to lose weight. I do it to be strong. To be proud of what this 'perceived' knackered body can do. I love my body and the life it's managed to give me so far. I will not take it for granted. Mind and body now truly connected.

Postscript: I can vouch for this. Leana does this so well that I frequently have to remind myself that she has any limitations at all. It is a testament to her mindset.

How to Change a Mind

This all sounds great in practice, but how do you change your mind? Good question. For fear of coming off a bit Professor Pumpernickle (I'm not, you'll see) let's go back to science and more specifically to neuroscience.

What If We Do Some Neural Plasticity?

Neural plasticity is something I love. I have no idea what it is. It's not that I've not tried to understand it. I have. It's about the brain and receptors and synapses and connections and I don't know – I've read multiple books in an effort – I'm going to give you my version, that I shamelessly nicked from Catherine Gray's The Unexpected Joy of Being Sober[61], she explains it better. Catherine talks about changing our habits and addictions (and our thoughts, assumptions and beliefs in fantasy bodies are habits) with regard to shifting our neural pathways. Habitual pathways in the brain, are formed '… in a similar way to hiking trails, the more a hiking trail is used, the smoother, wider and clearer it becomes. It becomes the default, easiest route.' So starting to think differently about ourselves, even backed up with clear evidence, on the first try, is incredibly hard, looks nothing like a path and feels wrong, but as time goes on the path becomes more trodden, it opens up and before long, it's easily passable – even the obvious choice!

Neural plasticity is at the heart of all personal change. It is basically re-wiring our brains to a new reality. Re-writing scripts rehearsed since childhood and quieting our inner critics. Scripts that have been reinforced by the world around us – like everywhere. Strengthening new thoughts, displacing old ones, making new paths out of a pile of brambles. A really simple visualisation of this is to imagine that the thinking that has always gone on in your brain, your belief in the fantasy body, is a motorway, five lanes wide in your head, made strong and clear through a lifetime of reinforced images, messages, comments, thoughts. Meanwhile the idea of the natural diversity of humans is currently an overgrown thicket.

Only by adjusting those messages, thoughts and comments, can a new course be set. It takes repetition, just like the motorway did to form from the outset of your life, but given time (and actually not that much) and perseverance, a new route is opened and a tipping point can happen. Before you know it, the thicket, is a path, then a road, then the council invests in some tarmac as they see the new destination is important. Before you know it, highways is paying people to move house so a new three lane motorway can be laid out. It is still competing with the old five lane one, but it is now a viable other option. That's it. Neural plasticity. Not a receptor in sight.

I find visualisations really work for me (you may have noticed), to help me understand intangible changes, so I want to draw on another one. I read a lot after my diagnosis. Books that I would usually never have gone for, I didn't need 'self-help' (except actually I did). I learnt about changing my mind. I learnt that the way I think, what I decide to believe, impacts everything, especially how I feel. And I learnt that I could change it. That it is a choice. It reminded me of a student I once had.

When I was pregnant I used to teach reflexology at a local college. It was an evening class and often people would arrive after a busy day at work. I would always start with a relaxation exercise of some kind to help everyone wind down. During one of these, I talked about the idea of having more positive thoughts. I remember one older woman saying to me 'But you can't change your mind, it just is the way it is.' Did she think we were all robots and our mainframe has been soldered shut? I may have slightly opened a pandora's box for that poor woman that night when I reassured her that in fact, we are made up of all of our experiences and as such we've sort of been programmed. We can in fact reprogramme ourselves if we want.

It wasn't until my recovery, that I had the time or the impetus to really start to look at how it applied to me, to my life experiences and how I'd been programmed. I really loved this process, I kept madly discovering things about myself! The way I think, my route to it, the feelings it created in me, or sometimes I'd trace it back the other way. What's this feeling in me? Where did it come from, what was my thought? Sometimes it was mind-blowing! So, back to visualisation. I remember one technique, in Louise Hay's book, You Can Heal Your Life[62] that asks you to imagine the process like 'housecleaning' your 'mental rooms'. Imagine, your mind as a building, a house, and all your thoughts are like ornaments. You can walk through and pick each one up and decide if the thought is yours or someone else's, if it serves you or not, if you want to keep it. In this way we start to change our minds. It can be proper sticky too though, can bring up some pretty painful memories so do it with self-care and, if necessary, a good friend's ear or talking therapy.

I've been watching my mind since then. I've started to notice that when I'm not feeling that good, if I'm on a downer, depressed, anxious, it's usually because I'm beating myself up in my mind. I'm usually telling myself that in some way I'm not good enough. I'm writing this in 2020 and just yesterday I caught myself doing it. Once I realise, it's much easier for me to be kinder to myself.

In Stephanie Yeboah's book[63], Chapter Five, you can find a really helpful list of questions to self-analyse, that would be good to use with this exercise, all about how we feel about our bodies, and I'm sure some of your own will come up for you too. Reconnecting with our bodies isn't just about changing our minds, but about something deeper, something more primal…

What If We Acknowledge Our Body Feelings?

There is another aspect of body intelligence and, in fact, diversity that we rarely acknowledge and that is, our *experience* of our bodies (stick with me!). How we feel in our bodies, or rather, how we feel our emotions in our bodies. It is an area between our physical and mind health, It's part self-awareness, part body experience. It's not, how we're feeling - happy, sad, grief, elation (although they can also be felt in our bodies) but how our actual bodies feel on a day-to-day, shifting hour-to-hour basis. What are they telling us? How connected are we to that aspect of health, to that aspect of ourselves? People can be having a stress response, raised adrenalin and inflammation markers without giving any hints away that they are.

Some people feel this very clearly, have direct access to this part of them, can relate body feelings to events or emotions in their lives and process them with skills they've picked up along the way. Other people have a very different experience of their bodies, especially if they've dealt with trauma as a child. They may suffer from a long-term stress reaction they themselves might think is normal. So they might not even be aware of their body feelings, or have ready access to them. Other considerations might be that some can be emotionally lazy or not give themselves permission to have emotions, or pay attention to them. These states and the spectrum of what must lie between them has a big impact on our self-awareness. As we all engage with it on varying levels it differs in each of us. How much we give it our attention and focus, is as diverse as we are. Some find it easy to articulate their inner worlds, others less so. It can impact how we process our emotions and whether they linger long-term and begin to feel just like normal and unchangeable, or whether we can harness our powers of body intelligence and process them more effectively. (There's a whole other book in me on this subject btw).

Are you ready for another hoaxy body thing? This is well-documented, under the field of study known as psychoneuroimmunology. How we feel in our bodies and its impact on our immune system via the nervous system. Dr Gabor Maté who is a specialist in trauma has written the book, *When the Body Says No - The Cost of Hidden Stress* speaking here on a podcast, he has this to say:

'... given that (for most physicians) their training doesn't touch upon that (the mind body connection), that's very uncomfortable territory and so they tend to resist or not to pay attention to that kind of research or knowledge, despite the fact that it's published in major medical journals and scientific publications.'

Maté further notes that if a finding isn't attached to Big Pharma, it doesn't get any airtime in the medical world.

'Millions and millions and millions of people could lead much healthier lives if this basic scientific awareness was infused into medical practice, but it isn't and the word trauma is not even mentioned in medical schools, for the most part...There are thousands of research papers on these connections.'[64]

Maté also points out that 'trauma' doesn't have to be violence or abuse, simply the internal result of something external. And this can lead to a disconnection from ourselves in trying to process emotions that don't seem to fit or be acceptable, in the world around us, like, for example a lifetime of The Glitch and us not being able to reconcile our bodies with it.

I will let you draw your own conclusions about emotions we try to bury and any links to eating behaviours... With all this in mind, you can see how it is another significant part of our life-experience that remains untapped, unexplored. A potential that we don't reap, yet could bring us increased health, in spades.

What we believe
Informs what we think
Informs how we feel
Informs our body feelings

By looking at what we believe, (for example *I should have a thin body*), and how it informs our thoughts (*I need to lose weight*), which leads to an unnecessary emotion (*I'm not good enough like this*) and creates a negative body feeling (tension in my tummy, wasted brainpower). We can also chase it back the other way and assess whether the belief really warrants the feeling.

You know, we actually give our vehicles more credit, by taking them to the garage at the first warning light or incongruous noise. We sometimes don't even know what our warning lights are. Pain, yes, or maybe just an unease that has been there since childhood, unchecked; or tension; recurring or stubborn ailments. Even if we do, we can often ignore them for years. We don't behave like our bodies are vital machines and need tune ups. The number of times a new client has come to me, having put up with pain for months, even years and expressed their surprise, delight and disbelief that I have 'fixed them'.

Or, the many cynical comments I hear around the effectiveness of physiotherapy. 'Ugh they gave me exercises but let's face it I won't do them'. OK friend, stay broken. It highlights generally how much we don't know about our bodies and how to maintain them. Body work, like mine, can often be given a voodoo association, something like witchery and figment. Essentially I am a massage therapist. I help people feel better in their bodies. I work on the mechanics to help the engine work well inside. It does require using energy and tapping into lifeforce – an otherworldly word but think about it – the force of our lives, the potential we maybe don't pay attention to. Essentially, it is still just mechanics, you just can't easily open the bonnet and see the machine!

My experience of working on people's bodies for most of my career, is that many of us aren't connected to this aspect of ourselves, it gets largely ignored, deprioritised, if we are even aware that it exists at all beyond – ow that hurts! It's an abstract concept - your connection to your body is yours and yours alone. You'll never know if, how you feel in your body is the same or differs to anyone else.

I love that my work, with the collaboration of my client, can neutralize these feelings. Install a reboot, if you like. Download the feelings that no longer serve us. Weekly or monthly bring people relief with the tools and permission to… let go of what doesn't feel right in our bodies. Still people would rather spend more on their hair!

And yet this relationship is the longest and most important one we will ever have. There is no one who is more under your care and control, whose happiness and wellbeing relies more on you, who's going to be with you until the very end, more than your own body.

And in wrenching apart the two sides of us, much has been lost. We pay it little attention because it is mostly intangible, we can't see it in our image-driven world, in our achievement-driven culture, in our status-defined times. It serves no purpose in the commercial model of the twenty-first century. As a consequence, we pay such little attention to our body feelings of: love for people, to the feeling when we laugh, when we hug, when we eat, when we orgasm, when we're lucky, grateful, proud. Feelings that could be focussed on, amplified, revisited (hello gratitude diary) and built on to create more positive body experiences and greater health.

I really became more conscious of this aspect of my body in the healing stages of my chemo rounds. More than just your everyday good feelings, through meditation and visualisation I started to connect with a part of me that feels, really, really good! I know! During chemo! I had never accessed it before, except maybe towards the end of a holiday when life's woes get put on pause for a bit! A sense of relaxation but also a connection to an essential part of me. It was a realisation that underneath all of the junk life throws at us – and we hold in our bodies – is this really spectacular feeling we spend very little time honouring. To me it is bliss and I could actually feel my body healing in its presence. It's what I aim to create for my clients and it is an authentic body connection.

Because our body experience just is. It is often seen as something that happens spontaneously to us, we take it for granted, don't engage with and perhaps believe it's not within our control. We just are it. When actually we're missing that it is an untapped well of positive potential and our connection to it can be healed. So how can we better tap into and reconnect to that? We can start not by just, not believing in fantasy bodies but by whole-heartedly starting to believe in something else, something more real, more tangible, more achievable.

Before I finish this section, it should be noted, we can very much ignore our emotional states too. On the subject of emotion, the transaction between emotion and how we feel it in our bodies, can go on a lot longer than the thought or event that triggered the emotion. If we don't acknowledge that, it remains. If we do, we can help to shift it. We can think of our inner worlds as a balance that needs to be restored for optimum health. Any emotion weighing it down for too long, might indicate a problem; is worth looking at to fix.

Additionally, our experience of our own inner worlds, can feel very real and yet jar wildly in response to the world around us. Our response to that can often be, to deny our own feelings. Sometimes acknowledging the way we feel inside can be really painful, ignoring it can be a form of survival, or simply we don't have the resources or the words to process how we feel. Sometimes the way we feel is utterly subconscious, we're not aware of it. In both instances, this can be painful, so please take care and speak up with someone you trust, if you need to. Some helplines are available at the back of the book.

So what else will help?

What If… A Mirror Is Just A Mirror?

What if we can see, I mean *think*, past the superficial nonsense that we all should be the same? What if this mirror is just a reflection device? (it is). What if it isn't loaded with meaning and judgement (it isn't – that's us, we can change, mirrors can't). What if a mirror, is just a mirror? What if we re-write our relationships with mirrors, cameras, filters (yuck!), clothes, changing rooms. Once we believe in an equality of bodies – of a natural diversity where ours deserves all the space it needs and a health we choose to define, this gets easier.

What if we wake up from our fantasy body coma, our body image blindness and really look, at ourselves. See what's there. Just see. Notice what role we perform in our family, our community, in diversity. Notice what judgement, rejection, criticism we feel and see that too, sit with the imperfection. What we feel we want to change, what isn't right, what wish we leap to. See it all.

Here's a task. Pour a glass of wine, find a mirror, put on Paloma Faith's Never Tear Us Apart full blast and just flipping appreciate your body. It was something I accidentally stumbled upon, but you know what, it felt pretty flipping powerful!

What If We Reframe How We Talk About Bodies?

What if we just stop talking about bodies. Ok that might be a bit weird, how about we frame how we talk about bodies differently. What repercussions might spawn from that? If we de-escalate comments and conversations about bodies. What if we don't talk to friends about diets, weight-loss, weight gain or exercise as punishment. Would we miss it? Would our life continue at a loss? What would that be and would it be worth it. Women especially use body shame (usually their own) as a way to ingratiate themselves to other women. As a way to connect with other women. As a way to bond. Could we bond, connect and ingratiate ourselves using other subjects? What might that look like? Sound like? Would more important conversations arise? We could talk about literally anything else. We criticise the male gaze and men's media for objectifying our bodies, when we do it, almost constantly.

What If We Change Our Compliments?

One of the pieces of advice I hear about parenting body image is to stop telling your kids they are beautiful or handsome. I find that so hard. I mean they're right! That probably is wise, but my surging maternal emotions undermine the logic and I could just burrow my way into them and snuggle all day. Awww my little gems! They'll be teenagers soon. Maybe it'll pass… So hard not to tell them that to me they are a miracle of eyes and chins and toes and elbows. The advice is, focus on literally anything else. You're so: smart, funny, kind, stylish, warm, talented, friendly, sensitive, compassionate... But more than that can we do that to each other? I've been priding myself recently on gifting random complements to complete strangers. A few months back a woman was alighting the tube at Euston Station in full ballgown regalia. A beautiful, emergency blue dress with skirts, drip drip earrings and in our passing, her getting on and me getting off, I slipped her the compliment 'You look very beautiful.'

'Thank you!' she replied and was clearly pleased. A couple of men trailed after her in black tie and I took the escalator, smiling, congratulating myself in my good deed. Except. Perhaps I was wrong. Cripes! What have I done? Is the age of the compliment over? Perhaps not. Could I have done it differently? Said 'I love your style' or 'You've made my day', which she had or 'That colour looks great on you'. Of course we can still give compliments but can we find something other than objectifying bodies as a conduit for them? Style, energy, personality, how someone makes you feel? I know right! It's a revelation.

What If We Become Body Neutral?

Unless you've been living under a rock, you'll know about the Body Positivity Movement. But what if feeling positive about our body (the movement is not actually just about that, but humour me for now) what if feeling body positive just isn't in our internal repertoire? Especially if this is a new path for us. Loads of people find body positivity – feeling positive about their body, is a bit forced, they *know* isn't really real – it feels fake - a lie. And it can feel like failure, another one. We don't *need* to be gushing to ourselves about our bodies, especially if it doesn't fit with long-term beliefs to begin with and aggravating more conflict. We don't need to be congratulating ourselves every minute of the day for being a goddamn Goddess (or God). An early skill to try and hone is just to pick out those negative thoughts about ourselves, notice them and squish them, like bubble wrap. Try just noticing your body, not yeay or neh. Don't attach a goal to it or you, like *I must stop being such a body bashing trout*, just notice it. I am a huge fan of not needing to improve ourselves. We're great just as we are, otherwise, we're still going to waste our lives trying to be something that doesn't exist. You may never want to celebrate your body or wear a bikini on the beach. Remember this is a 'selfish' process and what is right for you, is right. We don't have to be briming with #selflove but #selfcompassion is a must. It is absolutely A.O.K. to think negative thoughts, neutral thoughts, positive thoughts. Just promise to talk to someone about the ones that really hurt and leave lasting negative body feelings.

However in true contradictory style…

What If We Chose To Worship Our Bodies?

Not the same as being positive. Out and out worship. Listen, I looked death in the eye and it looked right back going,

'Yeah, I know, idiot! You actually need your body.'

Did you know at any one time there are a trillion cells in your body working to bring you the best health possible. A trillion. They reflect the many thousands of ways your body works night and day to keep you alive, to allow you to follow your passions, develop your talents, move, breathe, eat, smell, taste, just flippin' everything! Without our bodies we have nothing. Just saying.

Sitting on the toilet, staring at new stretch marks and a game of pubes on the run down my thighs. This is reality. This is my body. Well done stretchy skin that no manufacturer has been able to replicate. Thank you for allowing me to love people and feel love in return. For giving me stamina, energy, function, dealing with trauma in the coolest, most nonchalant sort of way, just quietly gathering yourself up and bringing yourself back together. Pain when I feel hurt. Illness to strengthen my immune system. Sparkly brains and their synapses, the capacity for neural plasticity (they probably sparkle right?) – meaning this journey has changed me. I have been allowed to change. The subconscious letting me know what I'm anxious about. The para-sympathetic nervous system going into healing overdrive when I'm resting. My anti-bodies, adrenalin, serotonin (feel good chemical), dopamine (reward chemical), oxytocin (love chemical), endorphins (pain relief chemical) and fingernails. And the ability to replicate this all again! Wombs and bits to make actual humans, feed actual humans!

Another gorgeous quote from Bill Bryson's book The Body – A Guide for Occupants:

'The body is often likened to a machine, but it is so much more than that. It works twenty-four hours a day without (for the most part) needing regular servicing or the installation of spare parts, runs on water and a few organic compounds, is soft and rather lovely, is accommodatingly mobile and pliant, reproduces itself with enthusiasm, makes jokes, feels affection, appreciates a red sunset and a cooling breeze. How many machines do you know that can do any of that? There is no question about it. You are truly a wonder. But then so, it must be said, is an earthworm.

'And how do we celebrate the glory of our existence? Well for most of us by exercising minimally and eating maximally. Think of all the junk you throw down your throat and how much of your life is spent sprawled in a near vegetative state in front of a glowing screen. Yet in some kind of miraculous way our bodies look after us, extract nutrients from the miscellaneous foodstuffs we push into our faces and somehow hold us together, generally at a pretty high level, for decades. Suicide by lifestyle takes ages.'[65]

I remember having a thought similar to this during my recovery, when my relationship with food became disordered and everything I put in my mouth was assessed for carcinogenic properties (another unnecessary loss). I had to have a word with myself and realised it would actually be really hard to try and kill myself with food. These days I will still be cautious about the amount of sugar and alcohol I take in, but I don't ban or restrict any food type and I spritz on my favourite perfume and enjoy myself whenever I want, no guilt or conflict. Those social rituals can be a sort of therapy. It did all get a bit skewed in the head there for a time.

Anyway, while most people wouldn't dream of skipping their appointment at the hairdressers (how they look), a massage (how they feel) falls down people's lists of priorities, even in the face of a multitude of physical benefits, not least making time for and honouring the most important tool of our lives. Vive la massage! Not that I'm biased by any means! But seriously, get your bones a good rubdown, as often as you can and remember to thank them and all the other parts of flesh and skin and eyeballs and toenails and nostril hairs!

What If… We Focus on Other Things?

There is a marvellous researcher/professor working out of Maastricht University in the Netherlands called Jessica Alleva. I made contact with her because Jessica is conducting of-the-moment research that indicates that there are experiences that both limit and expand a person's relationship with their body. Alleva's 2018 study[66] uses the tailored Expand Your Horizon's programme. This is a study programme where participants are taught how to develop body complexity - a re-aligning of their focus away from their body as an image to acknowledge the many functions it provides. For example, the body's internal processes - emotions and body feelings, our physical capacity – walking, cooking, getting down on one knee, riding a unicycle, those kinds of things, bodily senses - which it turns out are much further reaching than just the traditional five, such as our sense of balance or speed or appetite; our self-care and grooming, painting our nails, trimming our beards (bleaching our mumstaches!) whipping our hair into ice cream bouffants, and finally communication with others – hugging, laughing, snoggin' people's faces off.

Alleva proved that focussing on body functionality could improve body image by counteracting the harmful tendency to view one's own body based predominantly on its physical appearance rather than its functioning. 'The findings showed that the women in the Expand Your Horizon programme, who focussed on their body functionality, experienced improved trait appearance satisfaction, and body appreciation at post-test, and these effects persisted to both one week and one month follow-up.'

However 'Further exposure to beauty-ideal media imagery at one week follow-up led to reductions in women's body satisfaction, but neither body complexity nor body-self integration nor taking part in the intervention programme buffered these effects.' Women did find an improved relationship with their bodies through the programme and the idea of focussing on our bodies' functionality as a method to appreciate our bodies beyond just how they look was proven, but also implies we need to be on-it, virtually constantly to begin with. Alleva concludes: 'It could be that integrating the body and the self might require more time and practice (the body disconnection being) a perspective that likely developed over a long period of time.'

What If… We Relax On Holiday?

Holidays... the build up, the anticipation. The getting things done and the ticking off lists in order to switch off from life. The relaxation, the rest, the restorative sea, sand and sun. There's only one mosquito in the mojito... The body. No amount of waxing or priming will prepare you for the big reveal...

The immediate almost nudity in front of actual strangers. A scenario which, for most of us, under normal circumstances, is not our idea of rest, relaxation and general bon temps.

It can take a few days to relax into the new World of Holidays, no matter how many we've been on, because there's an internal struggle going on... There are the same thoughts plaguing many of us, I'm too out of shape, I should have worked out for this holiday, look at her cellulite, look at *my* cellulite! What does this belly think it's doing here? And it's hard to remember just how skewed and unrealistic those thoughts are.

We've been sold the perfect holiday (add it to the list) of mothers wave-frolicking or rakish girls rolling around in the sand, or the beautifully-posed sun lounger scam, sometimes women in duplicate, sometimes crossing legs in camp '50s formation. The truth is, there are sofas less fabricated than these wind-ups. They're the dreamscapes of marketing guys, crafted in stale-air offices far, far away. These holiday ad girls aren't switching off from life, they're at work, being paid... to hold their tummies in. And likely not taking full advantage of the catering van, unlike me, when faced with the international bounty of an all-you-can-eat-buffet! Because FOOD ROCKS!

So here is the truth you must hold close to you on summer vaycay. You simply can't relax and hold your tummy in at the same time. Try it now. Hold your tummy in and take a deep relaxing breath. If you've ever done yoga or mindfulness, chances are you may have come across full belly breathing. This is using the full extent of the lungs to breathe and you need to push out your tummy to do it, to expand the lower lungs. Pushed-out-tummy-breathing is a super-charged way to chill. It creates uber-good vibes in your body. It kick-starts the parasympathetic nervous system to help you relax, which also aids any healing which might need to take place and the digestion of that plate of prawns, falafal, gateaux and cheese you just put away. You see it's a win:win.

What's more, why not order a side-helping of gratitude for your body too. Is it performing? Is it feeling ok? It's ok even if it's not, it's still performing thousands of functions. Did it make this holiday possible by packing the many clothes you will and won't wear, but that you treat to far-reaching trips anyway? Can it put its own sun cream on? Can it embrace loved ones and create snap-shot memories to Insta (I mean cherish)?

So on your next holiday – especially your first post-Covid holiday! I implore you to breathe, not try and be thinner. Because holidays are for letting go of the usual strains of life. When I eventually get this body on a sun-lounger, I'm going to indulge in not-giving-a-flying-flip-flop about a bit of belly.

What If We Practice Gratitude?

I may have touched on this already. I was right to undo that warped *don't die kids* programming in me, cos here they both are, on the verge of teenagers. Thank you, thank you, thank you! What a loss to my life these last thirteen years would have been had I allowed myself to keep thinking like that. In the intervening years I have bought so many gratitude diaries, for myself but for others too. I've recommended them to countless more. I have no idea if people use them, it's ok (cut to: all my friends scrabbling to find their gratitude diaries, back of a drawer, under the bed). But I kinda get the feeling that some people think How can that possibly help me? Waste of time. Touchy Feely Nonsense. And that's ok. Gratitude has also been receiving a bit of a bad rap recently and I think perhaps if you approach it not as a reframing of your life and how you perceive it but instead as a method to be eternally optimistic and in denial of your real emotions, then yep, it's not going to work so well. I'm going to explain here though, how it helps me. How this one small act has shifted my perspective on life – and my body – more than anything else.

Attention. Without my gratitude diary entry, two minutes every night, I don't pay attention to good things. I might be more like the old me, bumbling along in life, assuming nothing good ever comes my way. Without it, even if I did notice a good thing, I wouldn't have put it in my metaphorical pocket and carried it around with me all day until bedtime, when I could lock it safely in my book. Without my gratitude diary, I wouldn't look for things, reflect on situations and drag the lesson or the luck out of it.

When I was a gratitude rookie, I used a format to find my content. I would note down what I had: achieved, learned, enjoyed and what am I looking forward to. And I would use a single year standard diary for this. Now, a Gratitude Aficionado, I use a five-year diary and you know why? That gratitude you locked in your book, you can bounce even more gratitude off it next year, and the one after and the one after that… In this way, instead of my body (which features heavily, especially my energy) causing me to lose parts of my life, my wellbeing, my self-esteem, it helps me to maximise all those things. You'll remember I mentioned Satisfaction Training and this is where that comes into its own. Being happy with what we've got. There are days, when it's hard to pull the gratitudes out of the bag. Those are the days when you have to dig deep, when you can think of nothing, it might fall back on needs fulfilled like sustenance, shelter, a shower, socks… or paying attention to how things could have turned out worse and we're reminded we've got a lot to be grateful for if only we pay attention to it. Don't get me wrong, I still want things, have ambition and aspirations but I'm also really chuffed with things as they are. As a few of *The Body Hoax* contributors have already pointed out, creating that kind of atmosphere in ourself, often leads to great things.

If you were to read my gratitude diary, it reads like a flipping fairy tale! It's the same life, just a different angle on it. It has made a happier, more positive person out of me.

It does however rely on me perceiving my relationship with my life as a creative tool, one worthy of my time and effort investment.

What If We Get Selfish?

It's not what you think. I want to finish this chapter by remembering the start. The power that Kim Chernin and Simone de Beauvoir spoke of and in doing so, I want to consider re-defining the concept of being selfish. Rather than it being something mean or negative, what if it was simply:

selfish /ˈsɛl.fɪʃ/

1. belonging to or relating to the self
2. typical of the self
3. (of self) having a very pleasant feeling and making you want to feel more

Synonym: personal, bespoke, individual, esoteric, self-careful, self-connected, internal crafting

Opposite: generalised, globalised, assumed, avoidance, commercial, burn out, external manipulation

This is the definition form of many 'ish' words, such as childish, stylish, moreish but not so with selfish and I think we should rectify that. For too long, we have seen self-care, self-centring, self-concern as being a negative thing. Of course if my children are reading this, there does need to be balance, but also, the true antidote to The Glitch is a warm embrace of the individual, an attention to its needs and a tender nurturing of the unique self. A woman in sync with, beguiled by the flow of her purpose, doesn't have the capacity to also constantly self-monitor.

What Training In Cancer Care Taught Me

There are two parts of my training at The Christie that help me in the process to reconnect with my body. We did a module called Therapies for End of Life and part of it was creating an End-of-Life Plan. Pregnant parents write a Birth Plan and I guess this is the opposite. It brought back a lot of memories for me. I had, of course considered some of these questions before. What songs would I like at my funeral, what type of funeral… This was a little more detailed and asked about who I would want to visit me if I was dying and under what circumstances. It was heavy stuff.

I would wager most people don't think much about their own death. It can be too scary to look at. For me, it was important to confront it. Shortly after my diagnosis I had made myself think about it. To imagine myself dealing with that news. It meant opening that jam jar in my stomach but I went with it. It took the fear and the power out of it. I realised that if and when that news came, I could mentally shift into another gear and accept it. I had to know that I would be ok with it, even though every fibre of me would resist leaving my family, I knew if I had to,

I could. Well I would have to, wouldn't I. But it also got me thinking, cancer takes lives, it's one of the ways that we die and it is awful, especially in young people. But also, a cancer diagnosis is a bit of an illusion. We were dying before the diagnosis, we're still dying after it, even in remission (sorry this has all got a bit morbid, but stick with me, it's important). All of us are on a path to dying and none of us know when that is going to happen, it's just as well we have these bodies that keep working day and night returning us to our optimum health! But actually with cancer, all that has happened is we've been forced to wake up, from a dream where we pretend that death doesn't happen, couldn't happen. Today! A pretense that helps us crack on with life. Cancer *can* focus our minds on not dying, on living a good life, when all of that was already on the table for us before, we just don't pay it much attention. And I get it, life gets in the way. Now though, I frequently think about dying, I update my death plan when new songs are released – Harry Styles I'm looking at you and your *Sign of the Times!* I try to hold it in my life going forward, because it's easy to forget that these bodies aren't forever. If you think that a cancer diagnosis automatically makes you appreciate life, makes you not sweat the small stuff and live a good life, it doesn't, that stuff takes time, practice and dedication. I meditate on death, because it reminds me how MUCH I have. How much I don't want to lose. It's sad but also beautiful. It can focus me on the bits that I don't want in my life and urge me to do something about it. I find it really illuminating. It doesn't scare me any more, I decided to think differently about it.

It really saddens me that people's last time on earth is sometimes filled with resistance, panic, fear, because they thought death wasn't coming for them and they hadn't valued their life when they had the chance. We must do what we can to enjoy our time. And sometimes that means having the scary conversation, putting up the boundaries, walking away, letting someone in. It can even look like looking inwards with honesty and compassion.

The second thing that sticks in my mind from The Christie is that it introduced me to the concept of the limen. It's a term used in psychology which refers to some kind of threshold or border between two places or stages – anyone currently in Covid lockdown will know this feeling! In the context of the course, it referred to the time – a bit like no-mans-land - between being who you were (pre-diagnosis) and not yet being who you will become. At the time I was still very much stuck in the limen of my own recovery, so it really spoke to me. But it was a word to describe an unfinished process, perhaps of growth or healing and not a concept I'd come across. Understanding that this was where I was, somehow made my frustrating endeavours and set-backs more manageable. And we can feel this on our route back to connecting to ourselves too. My advice would be, try not to force the change so much as live through it. Sometimes it seems that you'll never get to the destination you want, you can feel flat or confused in the middle, but knowing it's a process, a continuum, will help you will make it. Same for Covid! *sigh* Just keep going.

It took me a long time to figure all this stuff out. A big part of reconnecting ourselves to our bodies requires self-compassion. I want to hand over to my friend and Speaker's Collective colleague, who figured it out much sooner than me.

Body Stories
Sarah Hollebon

24, Fashion Designer, A Note to My Teenage Self

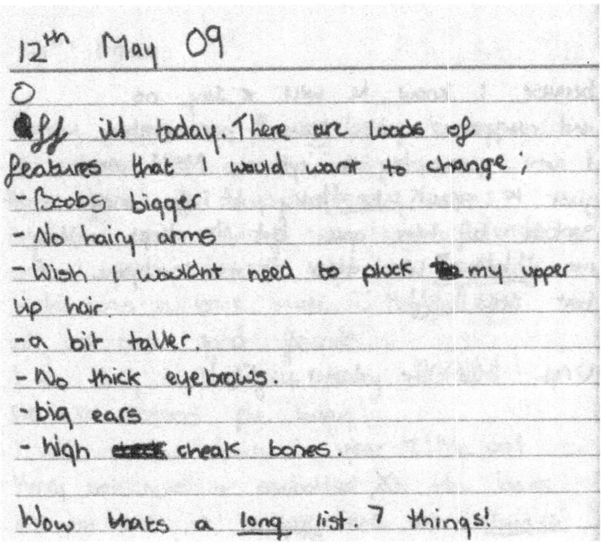

12th May 09

Off ill today. There are loads of features that I would want to change;
- Boobs bigger
- No hairy arms
- Wish I wouldn't need to pluck my upper lip hair.
- a bit taller.
- No thick eyebrows.
- big ears
- high cheak bones.

Wow thats a long list. 7 things!

Dear Sarah,

I'm now a few years older, and I've taken the time to reflect on your experiences through childhood and teenage years, and thought I'd write a few notes on what I've learnt now looking back on those memories. I hope these gentle considerations of self-kindness and compassion can help others around the world…

As a child and teenager, you felt it impossible to comprehend what lay ahead after school/college because you had yet to experience life. This led to you spending time in the shower having breakdowns, slicing your arm open, and wanting to die. I now know that sometimes we have good days, and sometimes we have bad days. Life is like the weather, there will always be a brighter day ahead. Please believe me when I say, life is so beautiful it's worth staying alive for.

From as far back as I remember you have always hated your ears. Ashamed and embarrassed of them. You got teased for them and went to great lengths to always hide and never show them. You would spend hours day-dreaming up ways to change them, pin them back or have surgery on them.

I admit I still feel self-conscious over my ears. However, I am taking small steps daily to become more content and accepting of them and treat them gently with self-compassion. My ears are a part of who I am and if I changed them to fit society's norm, would I still feel my true authentic self?

You put so much time and effort into making yourself likeable to others, you always forgot to put time in for yourself. Shower yourself in self-love, otherwise you will begin to resent yourself, especially your body and looks. Start each day by telling yourself something really positive or giving yourself a compliment. Affirmations are great for this. Looking directly in the mirror, repeat an affirmation out loud, once a day every day. One example to get you started 'I love myself more and more each day. I attract loving people because I engage in self-loving energy'.

You looked outwards for other people to heal you and make you feel better. Cease looking outwards for people to heal you. People will come and go in your life; this is a normal and a healthy experience for you to grow. You are the one person who will never leave you, so you should learn to sit with you, to listen to you, and to nurture you.

You got attached to narrowminded people who bullied and were unkind to you. You listened to what they said and took it to heart. You learn to ignore the noise from the people around you with the wrong motives; that these are not healthy people to be around. They are there only to bring you down, and that is their aim. If they don't appreciate you, then they don't deserve you. Please don't take what they say to you personally. It's not a reflection on you. Often when people are like this, it's about *them*, not you. You can learn to rise above them. You will learn to always rise.

You didn't seek help until it was very late and that caused you to suffer. There are people out there who will want to help you. It doesn't always have to be a family member either, it can be a professional or a trusted friend. It's a matter of making the first (albeit very hard) initial step to reach out, but it will be worth it.

You felt shameful and embarrassed over the harm you gave yourself and the marks you left on your body. Please do not feel shameful and embarrassed over it. Although self-harming was dangerous, it is what you needed at that time in your life. My scars are mapped around my body. A map of my journey through life so far. I am no longer ashamed of my scars. I was involved in a mental war between me, myself, and I. They serve as both a reminder of the dark days I conquered and, with the right tools and support in place, the future days I will carry on to conquer.

I hope these reflections help you Sarah and will guide you like they now guide me. I wish to thrive in my life journey and be present to the ever-changing beauty my body will go through.

You are a unique and wonderful woman, Sarah, and I love and respect you, and I always will.

Warm wishes and unconditional love,

Sarah

Sarah Hollebon, London College of Fashion graduate is a fashion designer and mental health activist. Located in Carnaby St. London, Sarah's fashion brand raises awareness of social issues.

Charities /numbers to call for self harming:

www.helpguide.org/articles/anxiety/cutting-and-self-harm.htm

www.youngminds.org.uk/find-help/feelings-and-symptoms/self-harm/

Young Minds also Provides free, 24/7 text support for young people across the UK experiencing a mental health crisis.

Text: YM to 85258

Progress

Emi: You know, I'm not fixed. I'm not healed from this. Insomuch as I still have flashes of those old thoughts. The other day I was shopping with a friend. Although I am not the fat one, she has always been the thinner one. We shared a cubicle like long-time friends do, while I tried on some clothes for an upcoming photoshoot. A long-sleeved top on, the flesh of my legs when exposed suddenly seemed… offensive. I think that is the best word! I saw my legs through others' eyes and felt ashamed. It was a millisecond thought that skipped to *I need to sort them out*! The difference here is I immediately neutralised it in my mind. I did not apologise to my friend or speak of my shame in any way. I didn't need to let her know that I knew they were not OK I very quickly remembered that they're just fine. I wasn't prepared for the moment, the full-length mirror or the ghastly changing room lights (why? Just why?). There has definitely been progress but if you're looking for total eradication of those thoughts, who knows if I'll ever get there. What I do know is, I much prefer where I am now, where I spend much less time dwelling in these feelings or thoughts or following them anywhere that might waste my time and energy. But also, it's not just about us, it's about changing things for our kids and future generations. It might be too late for us to completely rid ourselves of The Glitch, but we have a responsibility to put the breaks on for our descendants.

Postscript: I recount this story to my hairdresser the next day and she says 'But to me you *are* thin.' And there's the rub. We all feel this way. It's all relative. Just because a person has a body that you would like, doesn't make them happy and satisfied. We've all been programmed to feel less than. But also worth noting is that the body that we may be mentally tearing down, might also be somebody else's dream body.

For the last word on this section I have one more question, if you really truly want to stop believing in fantasy bodies…

Are you ready to give yourself permission to?

Because you are allowed.

Free Stuff!

To support this chapter and further arm you with the tools you need, you can download a work pack from: www.bodequality.com where you'll find exercises:

A 21 Day Body Diary – Breaking the Habit of Bad Body Image

Reflective Exercises:
How Does Your Body Support Your Life?
Measuring My Value
My Body Reflection

What Can the Rest of the World Do?

What can we do in our spaces, on the stages we play on? How can society Ditch The Glitch and Flex for Success? Starting with…

What Can Parents Do?

For me there are two clear things parents can do. Educate ourselves – we missed out on this at school, no 'media literacy' for us. And we need to put on our own oxygen mask before we can help anyone else. And secondly talk, and keep talking, have conversations around bodies, social media content, TV programmes, even if it means watching your kids programmes, just keep those channels open.

Here's my Speaker's Collective colleague Molly Forbes who is an authority on the subject of parenting and body image. Molly is a campaigner, writer and presenter specialising in body image with a particular interest in body image and children.

Molly tell me about your work:

I'm a journalist by trade and worked as a reporter, presenter, producer and researcher both as an employee and in a freelance capacity in radio, TV and magazines for 15 years. When I became a mum for the second time I started to really explore my own relationship with my body and educate myself about the huge subject of body image. It was only when I healed my own body image issues that I became aware of all the messages trying to drag me back down again – and in turn my own children. So I decided to do something about it.

I'm not a nutritionist, therapist, researcher or doctor, but I do have a talent for communication – I'm a good writer and talker! And so I set about utilising my journalistic skills to help bring some of the amazing work happening in academic spaces out into the public sphere, talking about things like diet culture and weight stigma and how children are impacted by these things.

Over the years I've been lucky enough to interview and collaborate with some amazing people doing really important work in this space. I was one of the hosts on Channel Four's body image boosting TV show *Naked Beach*, I started a podcast on body image called Body Cons with my friend (trainee counsellor) Lottie Storey and I founded the #FreeFromDiets campaign to change the way weight loss and diet products can be marketed around children. This year I launched a workshop for teachers and youth leaders to help create body happy settings for children, and at the end of 2020 I registered to become a Community Interest Company so we can create more resources and advocacy work in this area. The Body Happy Organisation CIC will offer resources, training and education initiatives to help adults raise children who love the skin they're in.

Would you say, as a rule people are aware of body image related issues?

All humans have body image – if you have a body you have body image! And we're all aware to a certain extent of how we feel in our body. But I think there's a huge lack of awareness around the impact that low body image has on all areas of our life – our overall health (mental and physical), on our social relationships, on the way we show up in the world, engage and perform at work and in school. There's this narrative that a bit of body shame is a good thing because it will motivate us to engage in more healthy behaviours, when research shows the opposite is true. When people feel good about their body (including children) they are more likely to treat it in a way that feels good. And there are so many ways we are currently, often unwittingly, perpetuating a culture of body shame that continually makes people – including children, some as young as three years old - doubt, question and feel insecure about their body. There's a massive lack of awareness about this.

Why is that do you think?

I don't think it's one specific reason, but more a mixture of many. The current narrative around health, the constant centring of weight in any conversation about health, an oversimplification and lack of nuance around what health is, as well as a lack of awareness about all the different things that make up and impact our health, is definitely not helping.

But also, the fact that all humans carry internalised bias, and weight bias often goes unchallenged and unobserved. Doctors, teachers, journalists, politicians are all regular human beings who all carry internalised bias and these biases play out in the GP surgery, in the classroom, in the newsrooms where the media we end up consuming gets made, and in the public health policies. Often these policies, news stories, education initiatives etc. come from a place of good intention – I don't believe anyone actively sets out to cause harm – but the lack of awareness and education around the complexity of the issue and how poor body image impacts us all is a real problem because it often means these biases get perpetuated again and again. And so the culture of body shame continues.

Can you share some statistics with us?

How long have you got?! Here's a tiny sample that give a glimpse into the extent of the problem in children…

Children as young as three express body concerns[67]

34% of five-year-old girls already restrict their food intake[68]

55% of 8-18 year old boys would consider changing their diet to look better[69]

One in five girls aren't raising their hand in class for fear of judgement over their appearance.[70]

You share a lot of great resources for parents, carers and teachers, what can we be doing to help with this?

I believe that change starts with having difficult conversations. This doesn't mean you have to be in conflict with everyone in your life or walk up and down your street with a megaphone and a placard, but gently challenging the deep biases that the people around you hold – particularly when it comes to weight and health – can go a long way. We have workshops, masterclasses and are creating a whole wealth of other resources, so purchasing some of these resources – even if it's just a £2.99 activity pack – helps us continue to do the work that we do. Also telling your school about the workshops or even signing up to one of our sessions yourself. Sharing my work on social media and telling your friends about it – all of this helps. We can't change the culture without having these conversations and the conversations won't happen if we don't recognise the problem in the first place. But I am optimistic and I do believe that change can happen, but it relies on a community of people being part of that change and driving it forward.

Where can people go to find out more?

I share all my work on Instagram where I am @mollyjforbes and you can get more resources, sign up for a workshop etc. at www.freefromdiets.org

Thanks Molly

What can Schools, Clubs and Academia do?

So beyond engaging with Molly's work, what can groups and the academic world be doing to help? Staff training and ed-u-cate. And by the way, not one attempt, ever, to try and counteract the flood, the tsunami of programming children and young adults have received about the wrongness of their own bodies. Not once a year. A regular / constant conversation and re-framing of our world to better reflect reality. This may mean training the staff on this subject. There are some resources coming up that will help with this.

What Can Doctors, Nurses And The NHS Do?

Do no harm and kill that BMI scale to death! Just axe it, get rid. I've not gone into great detail about how it was never designed for this purpose or how trying to fit our naturally diverse bodies into arbitrary numbers where 25 is good and 25.1 is bad, is just nonsense. Or how the way that society is distributed around the BMI scale creates a bell curve, the shape of which hasn't changed in a hundred years! Maybe ever, because we're… naturally diverse. I haven't done it, because it's been done already by many, many people but please read Anthony Warner's *The Truth About Fat* as it's the best take-down of the BMI I've seen[71].

Looking at charts of BMI although they have moved and changed somewhat in shape to show increases in weight, gradually since the 1920's they largely keep the same bell shape, most people falling somewhere in the middle, minorities being at the extremes. The increase, by the way has come alongside increases in height and affluence. It speaks of proof of the Natural Diversity of Bodies. Not that we should or even ever *could* all conform to one body type and as such an acceptance of our role in that spectrum is a more realistic and healthy one.

Equally problematic is the NHS's ongoing trumpeting of the fantasy body. They, perhaps more than anyone, believe we can all be the same. The Glitch is strong in them. I've just done a quick search for BMI on the internet and the first page is the NHS BMI calculator[72]. I input my real numbers and it tells me: 'Your result suggests you are overweight.' I'm not. It tells me what my healthy range would be before telling me:

> 'Your health would really benefit from gradually losing just 5% of your current weight. The best way to lose weight is through a combination of diet and exercise. We've got lots of resources to help you lose weight safely. If you're concerned about your weight speak to your GP. Aim to lose 8lbs
>
> Recommended daily calorie intake: 1610 - 2070 kcal
>
> To lose 1-2lbs a week stick to the lower end of the range.'

Could it be any more basic, reductionist, false, lacking personal agency or tri-ger-ring! For me weight loss has nothing to do with any of these arbitrary numbers and as soon as it does I shut down. I haven't got time for that! Weight loss happens in me when I'm happy, have a bit more time and space in my life, weight gain happens when I'm sad or really busy. End of. My relationship to food, exercise, stress, my body is just one cocktail of human of which there are many different versions on the menu. But it's not just about me, remember all the science I mentioned before about diets causing weight gain; about fat people feeling judged and marginalised leading to depression and binge eating? This is the service that is at the forefront of our health (and I am forever in its debt but…) this rhetoric is the blunder equivalent of surgeons in the early 1800's not believing they need to wash their hands! Wowzers can we do something? Further down the BMI page, after they point the finger at black and Asian minorities – not for their ethnicity having an impact on their BMI (it does) – but making sure they know they're more likely to develop some long-term (chronic) conditions. After that it talks about children and the scale allowing for age and growth – have you seen a group of children recently? Some of my daughter's friends at eleven could still pass for six while she could probably get into a night club! Not that I would weigh or check my kid's BMI anyway… or try and get them into night clubs. After all that and more, scroll down further… there is the statement:

'The BMI cannot tell the difference between excess fat, muscle or bone.

The adult BMI does not take into account age, gender or muscle mass.'

M-E-G-A C-A-L-V-E-S

Riiiiiight. Just totally healthy, helpful and supportive to have given me such a firm directive up top then. What's more, reading around the accounts of fat advocates, the shaming stories coming out of GPs offices and hospitals is enough to make your eyes water.

I've been trying, really hard, to make contact with the NHS but it's tough times right now in 2020/2021.

By the way, I'm maybe a pound into the overweight category on the BMI, and I shift around that by maybe half a stone. It isn't a gateway pound! It's not a slippery slope into obesity oblivion (scrap that word while we're at it). It's just where my natural body lies.

Here's my favourite point of Warner's where he talks about the work of Katherine Flegal, a leading figure in Epidemology. In a report produced for the National Centre for Health Statistics Flegal documented her findings of BMI and mortality correlations. Warner sums it up thus: 'Being in the overweight category with a BMI between 25 and 30, was associated with a lower risk of dying than the 'normal' weight category of 20 to 25. It even indicated that being obese, with a BMI between 30 and 35, still only had a weak association with mortality; so weak, in fact, that it was not considered statistically significant.'[73]

Still pumped off my use of 'thus' but also STICK IT BMI! I'm living the longest, how much more health do you need? In fact, research from Metropolitan Life Insurance data – you know the ones giving pay-outs if you die (so they'll know) - report that 'Thin people have more health problems and shorter life expectancy.'[74] Warner goes on to say: 'Perversely, many in the medical community refused to celebrate the fact that fat people were living longer.'[75]

In truth, I see it in my own family, my sofa-loving mother outliving my gym-going, Global Medical Director father, by eighteen years now. She's getting something right! She should be a cover girl on Health and Fitness, sharing her top tips! Just try and relax Pet, she'd say, and offer you a biscuit. Don't get me wrong, Mum is acutely aware of her weight and her desire to lose it is strong. It impacts her joints. But as for ongoing or underlying health conditions, as she keeps trumpeting after her latest doctor's appointment, she's 'Strong as an ox!' And if that weight isn't going to come off (and time would suggest it's not) I wish I could take away the anguish attached to it.

In fact almost all of the people I've lost young have been slim. The waiting rooms of chemo suites are not full of *the world's fattest people*. It must be the biggest glitchy world to live in if you're working in the NHS with a culture of fatphobia running deeply and yet not having that reflected back to you in the world around you. In truth we don't need to be shaming anyone about their weight. Definitely not if they're only a pound over a 25 BMI. Twenty-year-old me would have been horrified by that, would have stopped eating for a couple of days and then scoffed all the things before self-loathing myself to sleep. A little pocket of lost health, right there. Unnecessary loss. What a fabulously healthy process!

What we don't need is a blanket scare policy for everyone. What we need is a considered healthcare approach, for those people who most need it at both extremes of the spectrum. Which centres and gives agency to the individual, looks at their genetics, physiology and frames health in a realistic fashion giving them the psychological support they may need from the trauma that their lives may have endured. We can treat them like humans and give them support. It's so simple but, *ask* them what they want for their bodies, the most important thing in their entire lives, don't tell them! Christ! It's in identifying eating disorders regardless of size and for the love of God, stop blaming every health complaint on fat people's weight! Can we hope for a future, body intelligent NHS?

Sorry, that was a lot, it's just... enough with this now. It's not only starting to look silly but has serious, dangerous repercussions.

What Can The Entertainment Industry Do?

Right at the outset here I want to state that the entertainment industry features in my gratitude diary almost as much as my family! What would we do without it, especially in these times. I watch so much content. So I'm not anti-entertainment but I think a few tweaks and a bit of imagination wouldn't go a-miss.

During my recovery from cancer, I was desperate to find a reason for it and also for the sharp rise of cancer cases in recent times. (Disclaimer – I have not solved cancer!) But I do wonder, what if our culture is contributing to our stress levels more than we realise and potentially making us sick? I'm going to give you some examples from my viewing choices just this week...

- The comedian who cracks the joke that her favourite Chicago restaurant is the reason that, when she arrived in New York, she weighed 150 lbs! (The horror! Also, I am 150 lbs)
- The film where two teenage boys are in conversation, arranging to go to the school formal together but are at pains to make clear – *not in a gay way*.
- Or the house show that depicts the transformation from '*ugly house*' to '*lovely house*'.

My daughter at ten years old: 'That's not an ugly house, *we'd* love to live in that house!'. She knows. There are many women reading this (and watching that) right now who are 150lbs (and much more). There are boys and girls right now who wish they could be 'out' at their school dance and there are people living in comparable houses to the pre 'lovely house' who until now thought they were doing well for themselves (let alone those in lesser houses!), who on viewing these scenes have taken a mental health hit. Have been reminded not to feel satisfied, contented, validated. Who have been given the mental load of (a) feeling less than or (b) doing the work to remind themselves that this is a show, contrived for entertainment purposes - that no one actually keeps a bowlful of aubergines on their kitchen counter - and it's not about them. It's not even about the real world.

One might assume that entertainment is created for the masses - the mainstream. And anyone offended by it doesn't really matter, for the sake of eyes on a screen, or a laugh or 'freedom of speech', kindness begone. Inclusivity, do one. As long as we're speaking to the masses, it's A-OK.

Entertainment gets to feel ok and unchallenged. But who is mainstream entertainment? I'd argue that what entertainment depicts is a narrow minority of society. A format so ubiquitous as to now simply be set-in-stone, rolled out without any imagination to how we could improve it. Stories about white, straight, thin, tall, handsome/beautiful, rich, able people. Probably mostly created by white, straight, thin, tall, handsome/beautiful, rich, able people. But have you ever considered if, as a format, it's become an echo chamber of its own reflection – a echo chamber of mirrors! (I just made that up.) A parody of what people think entertainment is or can be.

It's actually not the broadest tranche of society, the statistically frequent. Maybe it's just who's in creative charge or at least their presumption of what we want to see, based on an historical blueprint. A format that hasn't shifted much in decades, but to get thinner.

In *Watching the English*, anthropologist Kate Fox acknowledges that the vast majority of English people live in 'a typical, undistinguished suburban or 'residential area' street, with the usual two rows of smallish, nondescript semi-detached or terraced houses...'[76]

The Independent writes in 2017: 'Today's British women are 5ft 5ins tall on average, weigh 11st (154 lbs), have size six feet and dress size 16.'[77]

This doesn't show up as visibility in mainstream entertainment. What if the whole idea of 'mainstream' is false, toxic? So, 'mainstream' visuals depict a 'minority' group - cripes! Could it be, what constitutes mainstream doesn't even exist! Anywhere. However, this mini minority group gets all of the airtime and attention. Yet, the common conversation implies that it's speaking to and for all of us! I'd argue, we're largely influenced by a very small, privileged minority and are left to try and assimilate our lives with it.

Entertainment too is body image blind. Real-life detached, repressed. There is scope here to really push more boundaries and create more compelling content that speaks to more of us.

Watching *Ugly House to Lovely House* (BTW previously named *Old House, New Home* – but maybe that kind of gentle marketing couldn't survive in a primetime schedule) my daughter is frequently outraged, and I have to keep reminding her, 'He's not really that disgusted by the original house, he's creating dramatic tension', (I say this in hope as I am a bit in love with George Clark, at least *Amazing Spaces* G.C. who, if he was to meet his *Ugly House* G.C. clone, would surely call him out).

In creating gripping telly, who cares about the millions of viewers taking a mental or emotional hit? Or that the format is a bit bitchy. The very fact I have to explain this to her, only highlights the duplicitous and disconnected nature of entertainment. You have to take your brain out, skew it a bit and pop it back in, to watch it. Probably totally healthy. Just don't forget to right it again after viewing.

What if trying to live a real life against the backdrop of this posturing nonsense is killing us, or at the very least, robbing us of our lives. Death by emotional pinpricks - it's a slow and almost imperceptible death! Making us work harder, feel worser, reach further, compete more to feel validated, unable to be happy, satisfied, comfortable, relaxed and present and ever have the hope of giving our bodies the chance to recover. And when it comes to bodies, unlike homes, those messages aren't just in specific home programmes, they're everywhere!

I think back to the average person of a hundred and fifty years ago. They didn't live in a digital, media-flooded age. Their worlds would occasionally brush with the upper echelons of society but for the most-part, they weren't concerned weekly with their: life upgrades, home improvements or directives of what it is to live well. Ah a notification-less life! They didn't know how lucky they were! They wouldn't get a carrier pigeon dropping them notes by the hundred thousand to let them know that Charles Dickens' new favourite snack was pickled oysters! Pickled oyster sales going through the roof… they just… got on with their own lives.

Just as I'm starting to think I'm being over-simplistic in my argument… when I'm writing and I find it hard, I take to social media for a break. Just now:

Facebook: Suggested for you: The Daily Mirror: EXCLUSIVE: *They saved thousands by watching YouTube tutorials and interior design shows * clap emojis **, alongside a before picture of an average home. I do feel muddled. So there *are* short cuts and budget routes to what the media has defined as standard (but is actually really flipping high). But on closer inspection, that's not what's happening... The couple had spent 50k to upgrade their house. This was packaged as 'budget' – The Daily Mirror has assumed I'm rich! It was still a fairly modest house. In fact come to think of it, that's what we've done! Quick! I'd better ring The Mirror!... Damnit! Suddenly I see our own home renovations as having been a pretty privileged thing to do. I've been sucked in to a none story again! EXCLUSIVE: Couple renovates house!

What is the solution? We certainly can't go back. Digital, media and entertainment are here and here to stay. The solution, I believe, lies in getting society into creative offices. Challenging typical hiring, casting and commissioning choices. There has been some commentary about the choice of Natalia Dyer in her leading role of Nancy in Stranger Things. Some have called out the casting decision as 'risky'[78] and a comment on Reddit from Jessyas:
'One of the first things I noticed about her was the fact that she had the body of a girl with an eating disorder. What I DONT understand is why the casting director would pick her for the role. :(among all the amazing, young actresses out there today- they must have had the opportunity to cast someone healthy. Whoever manages Dyer's career is obviously not putting her wellbeing before her work. Sadly, by giving her this role, the industry is sending the message that her disease is a positive thing.'[79]

It's hard to call it. Dyer may naturally be very thin. Either way, the problem isn't Dyer, it's the skewed perma-positioning of uber thin women and girls as role models. Dyer cuts a very vulnerable figure. Wouldn't it be great to have a raft of strong, commandeering girls and women in our influential landscape.

Moreover, we need to see fat people, not token ones, black people, trans people, disabled people, gay people, bald people, ginger people, people with skin disorders. All the people in all the 'mainstream' offices and listening to them with a commitment to visibility and representation. But beyond that, all the people, everywhere! Maybe that way, we'll see an end to the fat person always being the butt of jokes, portrayed as bumbling, lazy, dumb, having no storyline beyond a supportive role or one steeped in their weight and size. Kudos *Modern Family* and *This is Us*.

Maybe then we'll not have the current format of an all-thin fantasy cast and possibly one token fat person, maybe we'll see all the bodies instead. A real reflection of the world we live in. So that we are visible… to ourselves, not just for fat people, for all the human people.

Maybe we'll see an end to body-shaming jokes that are still apparently so acceptable, just today a whole segment on the radio, objectifying bald people. But honestly if bodies comes off the list of things we can validly poke fun at and laugh about, what are we going to make comedy out of? Anything else. Literally anything. And if it seems that as long as we're centring ourselves, it's ok to slag off our body types - self-deprecation is so cute, after all. But no. Other people are listening.

I haven't yet mentioned the music industry. In some ways, the most candid conversations that hit the mainstream around The Glitch, happen in music (see the suggested soundtrack at the end of the book for some great examples). However generally the industry is failing hard at this. All the fantasy bodies on all the hypnotic videos streaming into the brains of all of our most impressionable young people, sometimes verging on soft porn *is not nothing.* Film-maker and Creative Director, Ben Akers questions how women are represented in music videos: 'I believe there's nothing happening at all in music videos. Who watches music videos? My guess is the demographic is young girls. So for example Little Mix's *Sweet Melody* - is it empowerment to have three of them in bra's and Jade Thirlwall in knickers turning with her bum to the camera? Now what Jade is doing is obviously her choice. But what are the stylists intending? Is it freedom or is that how you get attention from boys? As a father of two girls and a boy I do wonder what we are teaching both boys and girls with over-sexualised music videos, not just Little Mix, but across the board.'

Sort it out music industry. Oh and gaming and animation, I'm looking at you too. And as for those body correction gaming apps, cancel them. Delete. Bleugh. Vomit… Sorry, I veered into fishwife then.

If you are in creative media and you're feeling distinctly uneasy about this subject, that's the right response. Keep going with that – until you push through your own resistance –until you fix it.

What Can Business Do?

I went out for lunch with my daughter yesterday. It was a hip place. All of the waiting staff were young, white, pretty and thin. This was an independent, off-street coffee shop in Chester, UK. What possible need could there be to employ the 1%? I could see that the manager was very slim. I wondered if she couldn't see it - was she body image blind? Did her body bias making her blind to the optics. Or did she feel that the optics gave her credibility, as they once would. It made me reflect that any business not employing a team with the natural diversity of bodies, does not have an equality mindset. Has scope to learn.

I experienced the shift I'm talking about myself when I decided to upgrade my website to include more body diverse imagery. I paid for the diverse images when I could have used free ones of very thin people. It made me reflect on why I'd chosen my original images years ago – all thin, to mirror the narrative of visual merchandising we see everywhere. It hadn't occurred to me then, to do it any differently. It had been about trying to portray the most appealing, traditional sales images and it was clear now that my values and beliefs have shifted to portray the most inclusive images based in reality. The ones that will let all prospective customers know, they are welcome here. It is a definite mind shift - I felt it.

There's also an opportunity to model authenticity in business. Here's an example, Lynx and Dove are two brands both owned by Unilever, Dove's incredible work in the empowerment of women is sort of offset by Lynx's traditional objectification format (although I understand things are slowly filtering through as Lynx are starting to have the body image conversation). What's more, in 2000 Unilever acquired the brands Ben and Jerry's and Slimfast foods on the same day, a reminder that it isn't a question of business' belief in a product, or ethics, it's just business, money.

Business can educate large groups of people – across the board (help with that later), but especially new recruits and managers. In her book, Flex, Annie Auerbach makes a nod to inclusion and diversity – that along with flexible working, it 'will often inspire more commitment from young workers today' leading to better candidates and better retention. She goes on: 'We need to be truly inclusive and leave the old boys' club and "in-jokes" behind. To make a diverse workforce feel included, we know we need to create the right conditions so they can thrive and do their best work.' [80]

Love your Imposter author, Rita Clifton, CBE talks about the need for the business world to change:

> 'The world needs changing, business runs the world; so we need to change business.
>
> To me, that means being more human.
>
> That means business people acting more like human beings who have families, partners, pets, consciences, pulses, even a sense of humour.
>
> It means stop pretending they know everything (and only talking privately about how they would really like to do more good if only they could convince their shareholders).'[81]

I've seen this in the business world too, back to my first job at the magazine. I think some people can cultivate an air of pretentiousness or real-world detachment in an attempt to bring a kind of credibility to themselves. But it's not very inclusive.

Clifton is clear that this is a point of successful sustainability, but, it's also important because it is the right thing to do. Not just as a tick on an inclusion checklist, remember inclusion is the *least* we can do. Mind you, if you are a 'ticker', education in this arena would also score highly for your Environmental, Social, and Corporate Governance quota and one for Wellbeing too.

I'll come to all of the positive and profitable aspects of a more inclusive and wellbeing centric team in later chapters but in terms of the bottom line, it is good news. Dove, Curvy Kate and Simply Be, are just some of the brands seeing a soaring of sales in profits following their commitment to a more inclusive / diverse format.

However this conversation needs to be happening not as you might imagine, just in HR or within a Wellbeing Team, it needs escalating to the Finance Department. Overwhelmingly business operates with a short-range vision with regards to finances with eyes only on this or perhaps the next quarter's profits. This is clear right now, during Covid as budgets for wellbeing have been slashed while organisations try and steer their ships through the rocky seas of lockdown. However organisations often miss the opportunity to *amplify* the wellbeing pound – i.e. receiving a higher return through the budget they set for wellbeing initiatives. Anglican Water has demonstrated an eight-fold benefit after centring wellbeing at work.[82] And boy do we need it right now too!

Further, research released in March 2020 by The Chartered Institute of Personnel and Development,[83] just before this virus really got stuck in, in the UK, indicates that cutting wellbeing initiatives (such as body image awareness for example, among many other fantastic initiatives out there) might be short-sighted

The Wellbeing at Work, Survey Report highlighted their findings of the impact and effectiveness of well-being initiatives:

(Figures shown for both the private and public sectors respectively)

- Better employee morale and engagement 58% / 52%
- Better customer service 16% 14%
- Improved productivity 22% 14%
- Better staff retention 28% 17%
- Better employee morale and engagement 29% 31%
- Lower sickness absence 30% 34%
- Enhanced employer brand 32% 29%
- A healthier and more inclusive culture 49% 57%

One final point here, if your organisation's Occupational Health Department is offering financial reward for weight loss (yes it's a thing), hitting a certain BMI or similar. Stop that.

There's much more certain businesses can do too, which is coming up.

What Can Photographers Do?

One of the drawbacks small businesses face in trying to better model diverse bodies is that for the most part the stock image sites that businesses would go to for their branding and web pages don't feature much body shape diversity. We need more bodies in stock photos which means we need more photographers to take more varied images.

Photographers could also start asking clients if they want their commissioned pictures digitally adjusting or enhancing. This is common practice even in family portraiture and not something that photographers are always transparent about.

BREAKING NEWS: At the time of going to print, online image library Shutterstock have just released a Real Bodies Collection.

Woo Hoo! More of that please, to cover all genres, interests, search terms.

What Can Authors Do?

Well, we've touched on this. Authors could stop trotting out The Glitch, stop reinforcing the damaging narrative around bodies. Authors could stop just casually dropping diet culture into their prose. They could stop reinforcing the fantasy body narrative and treating it like it's just the norm, especially for women.

And there's Bridget Jones Gate - A number of body confidence commentators have reflected on the messaging. On reflection, with c.2020 vision, the film is obsessed with weight, I'd say it is a central theme to the narrative. At one point she writes in her diary '9st 4 (terrifying slide into obesity - why? Why?)'. [84] I remember also that there was a total media storm around Renee Zellwegger's weight gain to play the title role to what is, actually a healthy weight and fairly slim. Let's not do that any more.

In contrast authors could be modelling much better messaging around bodies. For now they could address The Glitch, beautifully done by Sarah Winman in *A Year of Marvellous Ways*:

'She opened the doors to the balcony and listened to the soft lap of the river below, and as she did, she caught her reflection in the glass, and she didn't recognise herself at first and she gasped and she had to fight hard to keep those voices at bay, because those voices are so critical and so eager to turn a good day bad.'[85]

What Can Celebrities Do?

On a popular streaming platform, a celebrity talks candidly about her pregnancy, birth, and post-babies weight loss. The camera focusses on a close-up shot of her holding a half-eaten apple.

'In order for me to meet my goal, I'm limiting myself to: no bread, no carbs, no sugar, no dairy, no meat, no fish, no alcohol and (sigh) I'm hungry.'

Later scene…

'I feel like I'm just a new woman in a new chapter of my life. I'm not even trying to be who I was. It's just so beautiful that children do that to you…

Ok this is seriously a huge accomplishment, because I did not think I'd ever get back in my old costume and I'm actually in it and I can still move. I still have a ways to go but this makes me feel good because I've been sacrificing and working hard. Huge, huge, huge accomplishment, yeay!!!'

Later scene – voiceover

'In each of us, another woman or young girl might see a reflection of herself, of her worth, of her boundless potential. The youth need to see their greatness reflected in our eyes. Go forth, let them know we're real.'[86]

They can stop doing that. Celebrities can stop toxically talking about and attaching value to shrinking their bodies. Talking about it as if it is inherent / essential to success, something that has to be endured. And they can stop pretending that it isn't their unique and privileged lives that enables it. Celebrities, like all of us, could stop talking about shrinking bodies. Failing that, we can acknowledge that their lifestyles are irrelevant to us but we shouldn't have to. They are icons, role models for a reason. These quotes contradict themselves.

What's more, it's not this celebrity's fault. You cannot know what you do not know. She is born into the same world we all have been born in to, been subject to the same fantasy discourse and conditioning that we all have. And it's ok if she, or anyone, wants to do it. Their choice; keep it private. Celebrities do have the potential to shape minds young and old, it would be great if they also take that as a responsibility not to create skewed unreal or damaging messaging around bodies.

What Can Fashion Retailers Do?

Are you ready for another tempting overgeneralisation? Displaying ultra-thin bodies everywhere, has no impact on society at large…

Do you know what percentage of female mannequins on the British high street are below a healthy weight? 100%. All of them. Mannequins that display all of the clothes in real life, in the UK, couldn't menstruate if they were human. What percentage of male ones are? Eight. Just 8%. Well hello there gender inequality! Researcher Eric Robinson writing in the guardian:

'In 2015, we conducted a formal study of mannequins by surveying all national chain fashion stores on the high streets of two cities in England – Liverpool and Coventry – that were using mannequins. In total, we visited 17 stores and got acquainted with 58 mannequins, 32 of which were 'female' and 26 'male'.

'What we found was that all of the female mannequins in these shops had body sizes that corresponded to that of an underweight human. We didn't find a single female mannequin that was a normal body size on display.

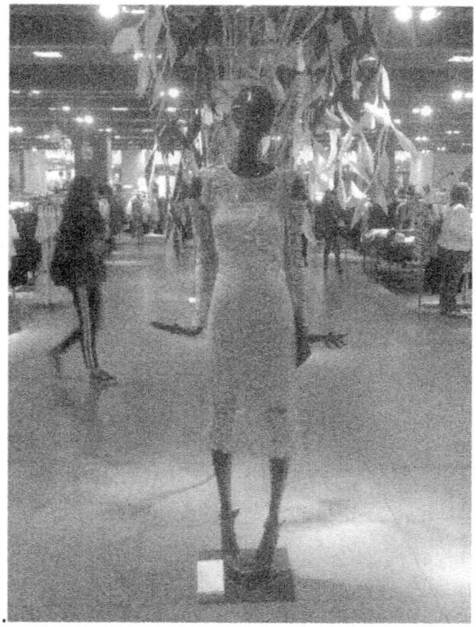

Photo Credit: M.G. Zimeta

'Promotion of the ultra-thin ideal has been shown to cause women to be dissatisfied with their body size. And, in turn, this dissatisfaction is thought to be one step along the path of developing an unhealthy desire or 'drive' for thinness, and subsequent eating disorders.

'Our observation of male mannequins show that there is no legitimate reason why mannequins used to sell female fashion have to be ultra-thin. If their male counterparts can be a 'human' shape and size, then why can't they?

'There is no excuse for the continued use of emaciated mannequins.'[87]

But there's more to this story… M.G. Zimeta is a Philosopher and Writer and reported as follows for the London Review of Books:

'Nearly a year ago I complained about the mannequins at the entrance of the ladies' department in John Lewis on Oxford Street ... Months passed, and I received no response ... The 'Fashion Queen' mannequin range I'd seen in John Lewis is produced by Bonami in Belgium and has the following dimensions: height 185 cm (6'07'), waist 59 cm (23"), hips 87 cm (34") and bust 87 cm (34"). A Fashion Queen mannequin is taller than the average British man, but with the waist of a ten-year-old girl in John Lewis sizes. Some of the clothes on the mannequins at John Lewis were discreetly pinned in place because the outfits would otherwise, even in the smallest sizes, be too loose for their frames.'[88]

Zimeta made a complaint, both in person and in writing and received no response. On a later visit to the store, she asked to see the manager.

' "A woman can't be that thin and stay alive," I explained.

"It's Head Office's Decision", they told me. "You'll need to fill out a complaint form."

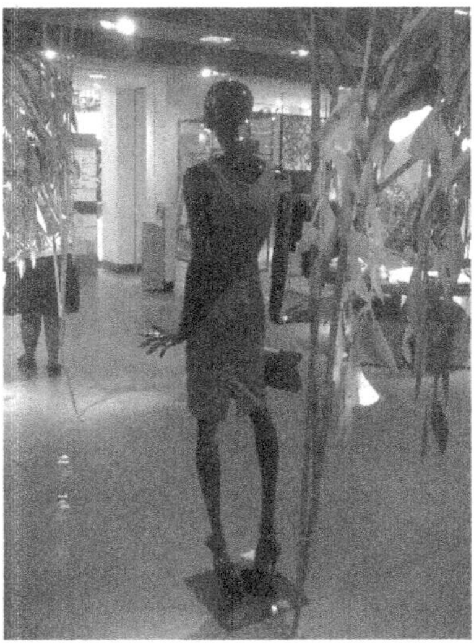

Photo Credit: M.G. Zimeta

This time I did get a response from Head Office. But they made a mistake: they accidentally forwarded to me their discussion about how they would handle my complaint. "The customer has said the first-floor ladies fashion mannequins at the top of the escalators in John Lewis, Oxford Street, the legs are thinner than her wrists," the Case Manager wrote, quoting from my form. "This is deeply unhealthy and unsuitable for a family shop. Customer had complained a few months ago but has had no response." The message was forwarded on, eventually reaching Communications, Visual Merchandising and Store Design Teams.

"I have the statement we put out re mannequins below," the Presentation Designer for Fashion wrote, "we tend to keep it quite brief as less is more on this side of things:

As a business John Lewis has for over the last 7 years has continue (stet) with a stylised theme , choosing mannequins for their creative visual effect that are not true to life form . Across all assortments of fashion they are sculptural in their look and feel . The mannequins primary purpose is to provide 3D inspiration, showcasing our Fashion assortments." (N.B. All grammatical errors have been upheld)

Less is more: a strange choice of phrase given the nature of my complaint…

I went back to the store a few days ago. The Fashion Queen mannequins were still there, in the same centrepiece display, in the same feeble poses. All that had changed was the clothes pinned to them.'[89]

So there's that. I mean speaking for myself, I always want to know what clothes would look like on a sculptured, fantasy, alien body. I find it very helpful in deciding if I want to buy them.

After working on this chapter, I had the chance to catch up with M.G. Zimeta who explains her own personal reason for feeling passionately about this:

'The reason I was so angry about those mannequins was in my late teens / early 20s, I was very thin and did a bit of modelling. But I was thin because I was depressed. And I often fainted or was too tired to do anything all day. I didn't feel comfortable sleeping on my side because I was too angular. It wasn't a healthy weight for me, but those mannequins were even thinner than I had been then. And yet John Lewis were marketing this enfeebled frame as aspirational. When I complained about it on the shop floor they said it was marketing for a target audience. I said 'I am literally the target audience and I'm the one complaining.'

Around the time the piece came out, I contacted the customer services assistant who had accidentally forwarded the email to me to tell them about it. They said they were glad about the article because they agreed with me.

Since the piece had been published, I've noticed that John Lewis have changed their mannequins, they look a bit healthier but I haven't measured them.'

I want to hear next from Advertising Creative/ Creative Director Ben Akers, who I met when talking to him about his documentary *Steve*, dealing with suicide. (the research for this book keeps putting me in touch with the right people!)

Ben worked in Australia for The Republic of Everyone, their tagline is: Doing good is good for business…

Ben: … which was my move into ethical advertising - an oxymoron, I know! When I came back to the UK, I started working with a company delivering creative solutions for Simply Be, Jacamo, JD Williams, not necessarily exciting brands but they can have such a great purpose.

I was working for an agency called LOVE in Manchester. And before we took these brands on they were literally, just doing photos of people turning around in circles. But we completely changed the way you look at all three of them, and the way that you attached to it. Especially with Simply Be. It was all about being real. The term 'plus size' makes me really uncomfortable in the wording when talking about models, to me it's just real.

The campaign that I did was called #SimplyBeReal and it was all about empowerment. We wanted to sell attitude, empowerment more than skinny, more than fearful. Basically my job is a problem solver, I looked at the original budget and they wanted four models in it. It was going to cost a fair portion of the budget for model fees, because when you get to these top-end plus-size models, they get very well paid. I thought, I can't waste half my budget on that! I happened to notice that their PR arm were running a competition with a modelling agency to create a Simply Be model. So I said why don't we work with that? Instead of finding one star, why not find four stars, we film the casting, we take them to New York, we put them through their paces as models we show them what it's all about, we support them, and we create models!

And that's what we did. We went over to New York, very positive all the way through, we put them up in a house in Tribeca, filmed mini documentaries around it. Created these ads. The first time ever and only in my career of twenty tears where a client has come in and approved an edit just like that, it's never happened to me before or since!

The client was absolutely amazing. We launched four jobbing models in their own right. We gave them a platform. It didn't just drive sales, Simply Be were also recognised in the creative industry magazines. It was a win all round.

A lot of brands are really scared to change the current premise of how you sell clothes.

Emi: I really want the fashion industry - and the advertising industry - to get its head, out of its bum and be responsible and ethical. Their refusal to look at this is phenomenal. I'm so interested to talk to you about your journey because I can't quite believe – I'm getting goose bumps to be honest - *you're* who I've been trying to find! I've sent so many emails, trying to talk to somebody behind brands like JD Williams, Simply Be who can give me another version of what selling products would look like if we did it differently and what the successes are attached to that, because that's what the world needs to hear. Why do you think brands aren't doing more diverse work? Is it just the money?

Ben: It takes balls to do it. It takes very brave people. It's like my experience of working with Republic of Everyone – the ethical advertising agency in Sydney, it was all about how we could do good. When I work with brands now, I try and find a purpose story in everything. We've been through the USP world - the Unique Selling Point, then the ESP - the Emotional Selling Point, then the Tech Revolution and now we're in this thing of purpose, we've got this new angle to look at stuff and go you've got a power as a brand a platform to create these things. I try and look at brands and say how can you use what you've got to change the world. I ask that of anything that I work on now but it takes a strong mind, a lot of guts, when everyone else is going one way, to go the other. The rules have changed so much now. Some brands are so far behind. When it comes to fashion especially, people don't tell stories any more. It's really sad.

In conclusion, can we acknowledge, that most stores and brands believe in fantasy customers. Stores could stop using underweight mannequins and pinning clothes onto them. Stores could take into account changing figures as they upsize clothes, not just make them bigger. Stores could stop erasing older people. Stores could cancel the word skinny in their garment nomenclature - a pair of jeans isn't 'skinny' unless the person inside them is skinny, they're tight, close, hugging.

Stop skinny washing everything! Take away the pressure. It's boring. Stores, *and supermarkets,* I'm looking at you too, could also stop labelling children's clothes and especially uniforms as 'slim', 'skinny', 'plus'. No one needs that kind of stigma at that age. Do as our parents did and buy a bigger, smaller age size (on investigation that's what they're doing anyway, slapping an 'age 9 plus size' onto and 'age 11 regular' garment!) or better yet stores, size kids' clothes according to… size, you know, cms, inches, and yes, talk about style/shape (narrow, straight) without alluding to size and shape thereby removing the stigma all together. It's glitchy.

All stores could offer responsible visibility through all of their visual merchandising especially their online shopping spaces. A day spent searching for that something special can leave us feeling anything but. Stores could get brave and try something new. The bottom line will likely stack up for them too! Funny how those brands having long-time embraced diversity – the ASOS's and the Boo Hoo's of the world – are currently winning more traditionally formatted brands Debenhams and Top Shop, in take over talks…

And finally, back to that comment of justifying the mannequins for their 'creative, visual effect'. Stop ignoring public health concerns in the name of creativity. It's not OK

You'll maybe sense my distress. The reason is this. The basis of work around The Glitch – identifying genetic markers, thought leaders like Jean Kilbourne, speaking out about the problem advertisers have saddled us with, started in the 1960's and 70's. Over half a century ago. Most of it consolidated in the 1990's – still 30ish years ago. And yet The Glitch persists - is a public health hazard. I am by far not alone in trying to break through to those people that matter, in trying to inform, educate and change their minds. There are so many writers, advocates, activists, thought leaders out there trying to affect the same change. Ultimately, I'm tired, I've worked so hard to try and instigate change. So let's take a look next at how it feels to be an activist…

What Can the Advertising Industry Do?

When A Woman Has Questions…

Put simply, kill the current format. Use diverse imagery, visibility and representation. I am going to make you privy to the inner workings of my mind, partly to lighten the mood of a heavy subject but also because, it's a technique that helps me engage with my inner voice, to work out where the opinion is coming from, to figure out if it serves me and if I need to pay attention to it or ignore it… Let us begin:

December 2017

Self-Preservation: I feel *very* uncertain about this. We shouldn't do it. We've already got loads on. For God's sake we're getting *married* next year!

Optimism: It'll be fine, I really don't think it will be that much work. Once it would have, but have you *seen* the Body Positive Revolution going on out there? There is a massive community just waiting for positive action. A petition like this is exactly what they're waiting for. It's not just *you* who's noticed the problem. *Everyone's* becoming more aware, mothers everywhere are seeing the impact that image-focussed media is having on their kids. They're bound to sign it and share it too. And isn't this precisely what social media is for? To take the legwork out of rallying the troops. For well-meaning change to go viral.

Doubt: This is going to end up just like *all* your other schemes. It'll cost us…

Ambition: It won't I promise. I won't let it. Listen, the petition probably won't even get published. Let's just submit it and see what happens. If it's meant to be...

Doubt: ...money, time, sleep, the capacity to mother, to work...

Self-Preservation: If it doesn't work, if it doesn't become an overnight meme and fly around the world gathering signatures like loom bands on a nine-year-old, we stop. Agreed?

Excitement: Absolutely. We take *no* responsibility for it.

Doubt: Hang on, what? What do you mean?

Ambition: Well, it's just if we petition parliament on this subject and it fails to gather 10,000 signatures then it gets thrown out and no one can petition it again. *Ever.*

Doubt: WHAT?

Self-Preservation: NO! Definitely not. You know how you get when you're stressed. You know how *Nusband* gets when you're stressed. You *do* remember the cancer don't you? This is putting unnecessary pressure on every...

Excitement: *Sorry*!

Doubt: Sorry what?

Excitement: I pressed it.

Self-Preservation: *Pressed WHAT*?

Excitement: Submit.

Excitement: Actually, we could really do with 100,000 signatures to get them to discuss it in parliament...

Also Excitement: Merry Christmas Everyone!

It started much earlier, when a friend on Facebook shared an article, celebrating the banning of an advert because the model was underweight. It lassoed my interest - there *are* things going on, there *is* progress. A light shining on a subject I've felt largely alone bemoaning. Also, in the run up to this time an advert from the

Advertising Standards Authority caught my attention. It went as follows:

'If an ad isn't legal, decent, honest and truthful, it mustn't run.'[90]

I kept hearing it on the radio and mulling it over. I started to pull at a thread and I watched it unravel. The knots I found along the way were surprising and have somehow (eventually) given me peace on a subject I had suspected was causing me many tiny, painful inconveniences: 'I'm not good enough', 'I'm too fat', 'My hair looks rough today', 'My legs are too big' and other unnecessary conversations between me and the mirror. Inconveniences which it turned out were obstructing my health, my wellbeing *and* my potential.

The first knot I found was on the website of the Advertising Standards Authority and the Committee of Advertising Practice (them that write the rules). I spent a few hours clicking around before I found what I *thought* was the cornerstone to the whole problem. The assertion that:

'...the use of thin models itself is not considered socially irresponsible.'[91]

Summer 2017

'If an ad isn't legal, decent, honest and truthful, it mustn't run. Our ambition is to make every UK ad, a responsible ad. *We* are the Advertising Standards Authority...'[92]

Decent. Truthful. The way adverts use bodies isn't truthful. It doesn't represent society. Not depicting reality isn't decent, it's false pressure and elitism. It having been a long-time bugbear of mine, I kept feeling irked about it and frustrated, finding the irony in an advert about the Advertising Standards Authority extolling truthfulness and decency, not being true (or decent)… Someone should tell them.

December 2017

I discovered Body Positivity or #BoPo for short, towards the end of 2017 and it was a heady flirtation those early days. Scrolling through Instagram, like a brand-new lover, it couldn't have been a breath of fresher air. It isn't just a handful of people thinking the way I do. There is an army, a tribe! Vocal, eloquent and bursting with chagrin. Posting images most of us have never seen before. Putting the fat body under the usual contrived circumstances that, until now, has been the reserve of the thin: great lighting, fab locations, posturing, posing, hair, make-up, camera angles, cool concepts, beautiful clothes, maybe some post-editing and photoshop … they look… gorgeous! Girls mostly, of all shapes and sizes. Smiling confidently down the lens, tossing their hair around, laughing, gazing, stretching. And like a new lover, to begin with, I observed with curious fascination. This new subject… it could be perfectly right or perfectly wrong. I kept watching. And I kept checking in on myself. The images were synced with captions that told me these girls were feeling great, and righteous and rebellious. They told me I could like myself too. And I'd been waiting decades to hear someone say it. They said it with a new language: self-love, body image, thin beauty ideals, love my chub, thin privilege, fat-phobia, body image blindness, body positivity, the Body Image Movement, body neutral and body confidence, fat activism, Self Care Sunday, Fuck Diet Culture, eff your beauty standards.

I noticed that my brain felt challenged by the images I saw. That I might see a photo of a confident, smiling fat girl and my brain would sort of flip and jerk. This isn't right. But I kept looking and felt the worlds shift like a Hogwarts staircase in my mind. Actually, this *is* right. This IS right. As time went on, my programmed gaze definitely shifted and I could cry fat tears of joy, because they are awesome! And their messaging is valid, intelligent and moving. And what's more reader. These folks sell some stuff! Their bodies are sellable. I bought a T-shirt from River Island, modelled by Fat Advocate, Lottie L'Amour. It's white with black, handwritten words on the front, saying 'feel good'.

Plus-size super models like Charlie Howard and Felicity Hayward, among a whole host of everyday girls, having a go and jumping on the feel-good bandwagon.

BoPo Inspo Infopics – a sample:
'F*%K thinner, eat dinner'
'Dear Self, I'm sorry for all the mean things I said to you'
'Maybe she's born with it, maybe she works on it every God damn day'
'You're not alive just to pay bills and lose weight',
'It's OK to not be in a constant state of self-improvement. It's OK to just be.'
'I'm not sad, I'm big boned'
'The fact that our bodies are different from each other is what we have in common'
'Weight fluctuations are normal'

I'm *so* glad this new place exists. Also, it's going to be so easy to tap into it and get my petition out there. I joined the party and invented my version of body positivity. I created my handle - *BodEquality* – you see what I did there? So obvious, how had no one else lassoed this concept? That like any other prejudice, diverse bodies *deserve* equality. I celebrated Christmas with an Instagram Infopic on my new @BodEquality feed, bearing the words: 'Joy to the World: All shapes and sizes'.

January 2018

The Parliament Petition:
'Require in law that branding/ads must show a variety of real body shapes.
The current position of the Committee of Advertising Practice is that 'the use of thin models itself is not considered socially irresponsible.' Advertising Codes reflect UK Law. The Government should therefore make it a legal requirement for advertising to show a variety of real body shapes.'[93]

The petition was passed. 2018 dawned and I'd invented a new, unpaid job for myself, and it *wasn't* planning a wedding.

Facebook posts:

8th Jan

[Do you love your body?] Well you should and could or at least not trash it. Outdated ideals about beauty need to do one! Who's with me? Let's hear the rally call 'BodEquality for ALL' I hope I can count on your support. Please sign and share - only takes two ticks.

9th Jan

Almost 100 people have signed it in less than a day! Could you be 100! This fills me with hope and optimism! I'm imagining these folks as a troop, a fairly big one. Prepared to say 'we want change'. We want to see all bodies reflected in our world. Please sign and share the petition.

The petition was off to a promising start.

Infopic Development General Meeting

Optimism: Right guys, we need to get our thinking caps on and come up with some inspiring quips to mobilise the *entire* country to sign our petition. Motivating, real, shocking. What have you got?

Excitement: I've been thinking about the Ugly Stepsisters.

Doubt: Sorry what?

Excitement: You know Cinderella's Ugly Stepsisters.

Ambition (placatingly): Right, what exactly do they have to do with this?

Excitement (expansively): They embody the advertising industry!

Ambition: O.K… *I've* been reading some Caitlin Moran and Emily Clarkson and I've found some great quotes we can use.

Excitement: No listen! Describe them to me, the stepsisters.

Doubt: Erm, they're… mean?

Excitement: They're not *just* mean.

Optimism: Well I suppose they're very judgy?

Excitement: Yes, anything else?

Silence.

Excitement: Are they inclusive?

Optimism: Well, no.

Self-preservation: And I guess they do have impossibly high standards.

Excitement: *YES!* Exactly, so high that Cinderella has *no* chance of reaching them. They literally make it *impossible* for her to go to the ball.

Self-preservation: It's a bit out of left field isn't it. I'm not sure it'll resonate with many people.

Doubt: It think it makes us sound too smart, snarky.

Ambition: (flips open Emily Clarkson's Can I Speak to Someone in Charge) Here's one: 'Thanks to someone deeming… that you were something to aspire to, we have been made to feel like our bodies aren't good enough.'[94]

Excitement (clearing her throat): Here's mine: 'The loudest voice we hear in advertising is judgy, non-inclusive with a perfectionist problem. Basically, Cinderella's Ugly Stepsisters – that's our social norm. Just checking we're OK with that #signthepetition'

Ambition: We could tag Em Clarkson in my post, maybe she'll share it!

Self-preservation: I think the Ugly Sister thing might come across a bit aggro, it sounds a bit whiney, dramatic, drastic. Might put people off.

Excitement: Oh come on! We need to make a mark if this is going to work. We *need* to be drastic! We need to make people think!

In the end both infopics ran. The Em Clarkson one got 20 likes. The Cinderella one got 32. Neither one was reposted or shared. The realities of the situation were starting to set in…

Facebook Post

14th January

The body image petition is bombing. Stuck at around 150 signatures. Which is a shame. I know the concept is supported widely throughout society. I know because I am a body therapist and the proportion of people who apologise to me for their bodies before getting on the couch, is steep.

I know that my loved ones don't love their bodies and it pains me to see/hear it. It isn't real. Only their reality formed through a lifetime of marginalised messages.

I know it feels *SO* good to change it.

I also know that jeez! There are more important things to be worrying about. Or not worrying about. Finding joy in life instead. Letting go.

I also know that this is not my responsibility. I won't own that even though I am *SO* passionate about it. Even though I feel my life's path has been leading up to this. *WE* have a social responsibility to challenge the current Advertising Standard that 'it is not socially irresponsible itself to use thin models'. *Yes it is*. It is socially irresponsible for a brand to use *ONLY* thin models. Which is our current reality.

I will continue to contact on a daily basis the many figureheads who are the turning point on this issue. I will continue to try and cut through the noise and the busyness of folks' schedules to say 'Hey we got 'em! An actionable, blogable petition that could shift actual change.' I will do it and I will enjoy it because the connections, the pulling together, however small so far have been heart-warming. I feel aglow with the potential of this collective movement. I won't stop my push forward with this. I believe it will be a success!

Diary Entry 14th January 2018

There's a lot of things I want to let go of: rejection, outcomes of the petition. I wake up in the early hours thinking *How* on Earth *am I going to do this*? I start to see how I'm giving up already, or really wanting to. I start to see how that blocks opportunity, stops me using my imagination, my intuition. I push through that feeling, it's still there. Very uncomfortable but I push on and promise myself to keep going, keep posting, keep reaching out. Feels a bit like emotional torture. *I want to run away*!

Meanwhile, something else crops up. I have a fear of doing too much. It's scaring me that it will affect my health and wellbeing. Then a thought strikes me, what if resting isn't my wellbeing path? What if action is my wellbeing path? What if this can be reframed not as 'this might kill me' (yes which is where my mind leaps to) but 'this might light up my life!'

I sit with all of these feelings all week and push on. The petition stalls at 150 signatures. Still I carry on. I force positivity, hope and optimism into my squirming brain. And you know, the week is a very fruitful one. I get offered two speaking engagements and confirm a third. This is all very good, all what I want. A varied life, doing good for society, being heard, making a difference. I feel rewarded, even just a little and it's enough to keep going…

Other Petitions

So the petition is up and running. More infopics are in production. I go searching for more inspiration and research to back up my case. I very quickly discover I'm not alone in petitioning this subject. Australian model Rosie Nelson has a petition running, hers is:

'Create a law to protect models from being pressured to lose weight!'

Rosie began the petition after being told by a UK top modelling agency to lose weight. After four months and losing a stone and two inches off her hips, they wanted more, saying she needed to be 'down to the bone'.

Rosie's petition (change.org) already has over 100,000 signatures. Oh. So maybe it's already in process then. I contact Rosie a couple of times, she explains that (at the time in 2018) in the face of Brexit and terrorism the government aren't really prioritising concerns that they don't deem urgent (such as body image) but that she hopes to get another parliamentary hearing on the issue. I'm curious how does that even work? But we're all busy and contact dried up.

Rosie's petition signs off with:

'France became the latest country to vote to criminalise the use of models who are dangerously thin. Those breaking the law face fines (up to €75,000) and up to six months in jail. And there is growing momentum for change in the UK - but we are still far from achieving a healthy standard for all models. The time is now for us all to come together.'[95]

A bit of googling leads me to discover that stiff fines and the prospect of jail time are now a reality. Not just France but other countries already have laws in place to protect models from becoming or even feeling the pressure to become underweight. They include: Italy, Spain and Israel. So we're lagging then. It also highlighted that France have passed legislation so that retouched images must include a label to state as such.

Then I come across an article… not everyone is happy in toytown… Robbie Myers, editor in chief of Elle had this to say: 'A law to 'protect' a population of what, 400 runway models? But it's OK to be a seriously underweight civil service worker? Or truck driver? This really isn't about protecting a class of people, this is about pushing back at an industry that defines beauty. I'm not defending the use of underweight models at all — my team and I look on in horror when these skeletal young women who can barely make one lap up and down the runway slump by us at a show. But you can't legislate beauty standards or legislate bad taste away, as much as the French have tried to do that in the past…We'd be much better off legislating for everyone to have access to affordable, healthy food than making models get a doctor's note saying they're fit enough to wear fancy clothes for pay.'[96] To begin with, I thought Robbie was a man, so entrenched in fantasy beauty was he and unconcerned for the female plight this represents. But no. Excuse my ignorance fashion industry. Robbie Myers is a woman… a thin privileged woman. Further, I disagree, we should be able to legislate against an unreal standard that, through its influence, at best is creating widespread mental health problems and at worst, killing people. (Remember, anorexia has a higher mortality rate than any other mental illness.[97])

More commentators pitch in. Oliviero Toscani is the Italian photographer behind controversial anti-anorexia campaign for Nolita in 2007 - the images are harrowing - the featured model and actress Isabelle Caro died in 2010. Toscani said the changes are pointless: 'How will it work? You can always say: 'She was 10 pounds more when she was booked." He also said about the retouched photographs ruling: 'All photos are retouched. Not [just] Photoshop, but even the way we use light can alter the appearance [of a model].'[98]

So there's a lot of resistance. A lot of stuck in The Glitch thinking. The point is to shift the culture so the model doesn't feel the *need* to lose the extra ten pounds. Yes we can't control every aspect of modelling behaviour, but we could state our standards and expectations for an industry that has a history and scientific evidence of widespread damage. Attitudes need to shift. It may take generations (it already has) but that's not a reason to stay stuck and toxic.

My searching means I alight on another petition. This one dates back to 2009 and the figure-head is body image guru Gok Wan. Gok's quest is to integrate body confidence lessons into all schools. He took 45,000 signatures to Downing Street, asking then Education Secretary, Ed Balls to integrate body confidence lessons into the Personal, Social and Health Education syllabus. Brilliant! Great idea. Except that was twelve years ago and body confidence lessons are still not an essential module of the national curriculum and you know… it's Gok!

The *How To Look Good Naked* host said: 'We need to teach the next generation that what we see in the media is not a fair representation of the real body.'[99] His co-campaigner, Shona Collins is winner of 2008 series *Miss Naked Beauty*: 'It was shocking to me how depressed and down young girls are about their appearance and body shapes. I discussed with classes how they think it could be changed and the idea came about to include a lesson on body confidence in the PSHE curriculum.'[100] All was not lost from Gok's petition. Awareness *was* raised.

Next stop, a convo with Credos, the UK advertising industry's think tank. My contact assures me the only way things will change, is through consumer pressure - in case you're wondering, that's you, me and us. Which we can do with gumption, petition and law-change. We have to tell them what we want! Maybe a shopping strike (I shall pop that on the 'to-do' list). Or favouring shops that have equality in their models' body shapes – Oh… but such places don't exist on the high street. In these times brands need to shout out loud to be heard, to make you feel an emotion, create a lasting impression, more now than ever. And thankfully, some really heart-warming messages are starting to trickle through that big-up reality, but this new ground is shaky and uncertain. Take for example match.com's *Love your Imperfections* campaign which I *so* loved back in 2016. The ethos behind it was inclusive and real and I felt good watching it. I later discovered, not everyone did though and the ad was criticised and pulled for implying that having freckles was an imperfection.

I'm sure advertisers (and the ASA for that matter) feel as though they're in a vortex of not knowing which way to step. But can you see the irony of the social problem? Society has been programmed to fantasy. So that if they see themselves in an 'imperfect' (real) way, they freak out and well-meaning ads are pulled. The ad should have been upheld in my opinion.

Dove are bringing supportive messages with their *Beauty On Your Own Terms* campaign and M&S's *Spend it Well* and *This Girl Can* messages hit a positive tone. Contemporary standards *are* starting to shift at a societal level and can hopefully pave the way for other brands to catch on and follow.

More heartening news, Instagram has attached support nets on searches including #thighgap #anorexia and #eatingdisorder, hashtags which trigger a message to encourage the viewer to consider their search:

'We've hidden posts for #thighgap to protect our community from content that may encourage behaviour that can cause harm and even lead to death.'

You can still see the posts but it gives you room for pause on the way.

February 2018

After many attempts to garner high profile online support, the petition gains support from long-time fashion commentator, Caryn Franklin, on Twitter: 'Signed. An excellent idea.'

Meanwhile, I discover Media Smart:

'Welcome to Media Smart. We are the non-profit education programme from the advertising industry. Our mission is to ensure that every child in the UK, aged 7 – 16, can confidently navigate the media they consume including being able to identify, interpret and critically evaluate all forms of advertising.

Media Smart provides free teaching resources and parent guides on subjects like social media, body image and influencer marketing. Join the thousands of UK teachers that have been using our media literacy materials since 2002…'[101]

So there are initiatives in the pipeline. It's really heartening. I email Media Smart in the hope that I can set up a meeting for the next time I'm in London. They may be able to help me understand more about why we feel the way we do about our bodies.

Awkward Conversations — In Conversation with the Advertising Standards Authority

March 2018: I organised a call. I explained that I wanted to find out more about what the ASA was doing around body image and how bodies are depicted through advertising. That my opinion was that the current approach is harmful. My contact, although sympathetic to the subject, affirmed that it was very unlikely to change. That it would be very unusual to instruct or legislate on advertising practice. That the current approach leaves room for 'free speech' and 'self-regulation'.

My contact explained, the difference between the ASA – the Advertising Standards Authority and the Committee of Advertising Practice. Lifted from their website here: 'The Committee of Advertising Practice (CAP) is the sister organisation of the ASA and is responsible for writing the Advertising Codes. The ASA and CAP are committed to regulating in a way that is transparent, proportionate, targeted, evidence-based, consistent and accountable.'[102] CAP is the advertising industry-facing side. They write the codes or guidance for advertisers to adhere to. It is a self-regulatory system. It regulates *itself* – more on this later.

I asked, what circumstances do trigger codes being changed. Have they ever? Yes, in the case of tobacco. After decades of research the link from smoking to cancer was undeniable. It impacted people's ability to work, it reflected a cost to the NHS and an economic burden. The tipping point came when it became clear, there was no safe way to smoke. Coupled with the loss of productivity in the workplace, it was deemed unacceptable to advertise tobacco any more. So that *did* change at a policy level.

I asked, out of interest, has there ever been any research into the cost of eating disorders to the NHS?

No.

(Incidentally, the estimated cost of eating disorders to the economy is £16.8bn per year[103], including: 'PwC estimated in 2015 that eating disorders cost the NHS £4.6 billion.'[104] More on why this is relevant later, if it's not abundantly obvious.)

They went on...The ASA *reflects* social change (you, me and us again), they don't enforce it. It would be inappropriate for the ASA to engineer society. Take perfume adverts for example, the image associated with that glamour is unlikely to change... (Emi: Only if we stay stuck in fantasy mindsets it won't! Surely you don't have to have that much of a progressive mind to be able to conjure up a variation on a theme, where diversity is better represented and could be classed as glamour. By the way, the fragrance advertising industry *is* lagging way behind on this issue.)

We finished our conversation that day with them providing me with some really great contacts to follow up with. They also informed me that there was an open consultation underway, coming in May/June 2018 which will be looking at gender stereotypes and body image would be one of the six subjects covered. This didn't really please me because the issue is no longer gender specific, although women have historically been more loaded with body image pressure. The market is now shifting to target men for their untapped economic potential and body image dissatisfaction is on the rise among them too. I asked to be kept informed and made a personal decision to respond.

An Inconvenient Truth

Going back to these stats for a moment... The cost of eating disorders is estimated at £4.6 billion to the NHS. Just for comparison, what are the costs of obesity to the NHS? Various estimates agree it lies somewhere between £5.1 and £6.1 billion (during a comparable timeframe of 2016/7). However researcher Melissa Owens highlights that '...these estimates are not balanced cost-benefit analyses. The costs saved on pensions, healthcare, and other benefits from the 7.1% of early deaths attributable to overly high BMIs are calculated at £3.6 billion per year, which brings the net costs on the state of overweight and obesity down to £2.47 billion.' [105]

While I'd never advocate for early deaths to save money, and I acknowledge trying to assess the financial impact of both extremes is rather messy and not clear cut, this does sort of frame 'The Obesity Crisis' slightly differently. It contributes again to a skewed narrative around bodies – and our perceived 'wrongness' of them.

International Women's Day – 8th March 2018

At an event held at Chester University, in association with Department of Gender Studies. I meet feminist and author of *The Beauty Myth* Naomi Wolf and quickly get the chance to talk through my petition with her. Her advice? In her experience petitions don't work. Lobbying does. Oh.

April 2018

I am suitably impressed with this! Not only has Mike Amesbury MP, supported the campaign. He has done his research which to me shows his level of commitment. With his permission I share his post and our communications.

Facebook: Mike Amesbury, MP:

'I recently met a truly inspirational constituent at my surgery in Northwich.

Emi Howe is campaigning to change how the media and fashion industries portray body image.

She started her campaign after having a mastectomy for breast cancer, starting a blog about her experience and setting out to encourage others to love and celebrate their bodies, even if it doesn't conform to the very narrow 'ideal' that we see depicted so often now.

Emi is a young mum and has also raised much-needed money for charity and is continuing to try and change not only how people are viewed and depicted in the media, but also how they view themselves - a really important goal that I said I'll be only too happy to help support.

One way of doing that is through things like this (publicity on social media) but I'll also be writing to the government and tabling questions in Parliament to try and get Emi's campaign all the help and attention I can. She has also launched a petition which can be signed at: https://petition.parliament.uk/petitions/208103

Dear Ms Howe

Thank you again for coming to see me at my recent surgery in Northwich. I am in complete agreement with your views and support what you're trying to achieve.

I have now raised the very valid points we discussed with the Women and Equalities Minister, and also with my Labour colleague and Shadow Secretary of State for Women and Equalities. Please find attached the letter's I have sent.

I will also be raising a parliamentary question on the issue and will continue to look for ways I can help you gain more publicity for your campaign. I will be in touch once I have received responses.

Best wishes for now

Yours sincerely

Mike Amesbury, Labour MP for Weaver Vale, House of Commons

The Research Begins…

- More than 100 studies have demonstrated the links between negative body image and the media. They also provide evidence that body image dissatisfaction impacts disordered eating. [106, 107]

- '…ample empirical research is available documenting associations between idealised images of female (and increasingly male) beauty and negative effects on women's physical, psychological, and social well-being.' [108]

'…negative body image has been considered a public health concern.'[109]

- 'People are often unaware – and mass media work hard to keep it that way – of the extent to which, and just exactly how (they) play an important role in promoting consumerism, body objectification and internalisation of the current beauty ideal.' (López-Guimerà et al, 2010[110])

- '50% of girls report being dissatisfied with their bodies, regardless of size.' [111]

- Among leading sources of disability among young women, eating disorders are among the top ten and of all mental disorders, anorexia reflects the highest mortality rate.[112]

- '55% of children have been bullied about their appearance 40% of these experienced bullying at least once a week.'[113]

I submitted a letter to the offices of the ASA informing them of their responsibility and highlighting the contradiction: The Codes of Advertising Practice, which informs the UK Advertising Standards Authority, are not doing their job. The ASA's purpose states that:

'Our mission is to make every UK ad a responsible ad.'[114] My assessment of the ASA's focus, however, was that in practice the concept of "responsibility" was being interpretated far too narrowly and was, as a result, completely missing the point when it comes to body image in advertising.

As an authority of standards, for CAP and the ASA to achieve their aim of "responsible" ads they must consider that concept from all perspectives; by focusing primarily on responding to what those who are sufficiently motivated to complain consider to be misleading or offensive, they are missing a huge element of their own aim. As we are all impacted by The Glitch, it isn't surprising that we aren't complaining about adverts that perpetuate it. We have been conditioned to expect it. So if the ASA is just led purely by what gets complained about, then it risks failing to regulate an issue that it, as the standards authority, should take some responsibility for.

And I start to get really frustrated. This research is literally the tip of the iceberg of what's out there. This conversation is going on in many places. Why are we doing nothing about it? Why do we think, this is 'not our problem'?

An impossible standard has been set.

Why are we continuing to entertain a warped sense of reality based on fantasy?

Activism
April 30th 2018

I hosted a screening of the documentary The Illusionists. It's a fascinating spotlight on commercialism and its role in creating insecurities and from that, a market for… just about anything. Afterwards I hosted a conversational-style panel alongside Professor Emma Rees, Programme Lead on the MSc for Gender Studies at Chester University, and keen supporter of my campaign.

A question came from the audience: 'What if body positivity doesn't seem possible?' It can be a stretch too far, especially if you've lived a life of thin-programming and self-rejection.

Emma's reply, 'Maybe we can consider instead, being body neutral?'

It was a really good point and felt much more achievable. It was a small distinction but somewhat of a revelation.

May 6th 2018

700 signatures

Ambition: Ok what's next? What can we do to raise the profile of the campaign?

Self-preservation: How about trying to engage some more influencers?

Doubt: We don't have any money. To pay them.

Ambition: Hang on… we're missing something, where's Excitement?

In a broom cupboard...

Excitement: Stop it, get off. I've said I'm SORRY.

Panic: You don't seem to have grasped the situation though.

Excitement: I do, I do, you're very… upset.

Panic: I'm not just upset, you've landed us in it again, we haven't enough time, we'll never manage it. It's your fault!

Fear: Fail. Fail. Fail.

Excitement (crying): I know, I know but what can I do now?

Panic: Nothing, exactly! Just leave us to try and sort it out.

Excitement: I promise I'll never do this again. I'll stop. I won't make any… what did you call them?

Panic: Unilateral decisions.

Excitement: …unilateral decisions. Life will be totally calm.

Fear: If we're *even* still alive!

Excitement: I still think though, let's not give up yet. We've still got two months.

Panic: Well we're staying around to oversee it.

Fear: You're a loose cannon!

Excitement: OK just try not to… interfere!

Body Equality in Bikini Shopping

A Blog posted April 2018

Recently I've been shopping for a new bikini for my up-coming honeymoon - eeek!

For a girl making strides in the world of body equality, this is a fairly sobering experience.

Regarding this campaign, where I would like to see ALL body shapes reflected in advertising and branding, I hear 'Things are changing', a lot. And they are, like if snails were in change. I do know there is fear... the bold move is, well it's for the bold and a mistake on this level could cost a business big! And make key marketing folks look pretty silly in the process, maybe even cost them their jobs! Any Marketing Exec willing to stick their neck out and re-write the rules about how to sell clothes, is gonna have to be an epic individual with almost super-human capabilities. This is one of the reasons why diversity in ads should be mandatory. Did I mention my petition?

- ASOS is by far the market leader, trail-blazer and enlightened thinker in this department. Last week model Vivian Eyo-Ephraim lit up social media with a shoot she did for ASOS. They have also stopped airbrushing their photos as of last year and their clear commitment to moving forward on this issue is truly commendable. Top Marks!

- John Lewis I liked because they nonchalantly just dropped the curves in there, no pomp and circumstance, not *ta da - here's the big girls clothes!* I found diverse bodies just moseying on around with the fantasy models.
- Very, actually perform much like ASOS, the curves are there, but you have to search for them.
- Debenhams did OK... and I found Curvy Kate on page one. I mean it's by no means enough but a nod to progress, I wonder if it slipped in in error because there wasn't another plus size model until page six...
- New Look's curves also featured fairly early on.
- National treasure, M&S came out badly in this, no diversity at all on their bikini page. Which surprises me as they showed their commitment to diversity through the launch of their Curve range earlier this year. Not in swimwear though.
- Next - You literally have to scroll through hundreds of images of idealised bodies to reach the section for Curvy Kate and Pour Moi. They are there, way down, no keep going, out the back, behind the bins.... The images generally are also the most contrived in terms of posing. Those girls are not breathing!
- Primark do something different. They remove the bodies all together. I've noticed H&M do this and M&S doing it in some of their other ranges too. I like it, makes it purely about the product!
- Adidas - no diversity - but not the traditional idealised body, the models were all athletic. Different, not better.
- Zara, I think while being racially centric, are not diverse at all on body shape.

Looking at other online companies I've previously used: Hush, The White Company, don't even go there... no diversity, in shape, ethnicity, poses more contrived. They are definitely the underdogs at this game and, to my eyes anyway, this kind of branding is starting to look really dated.

In summary yes, things are changing, but piecemeal and slower than a sloth on a hot day. The idealised body accounts for the natural body shape of five per cent of the population. With these forward moves maybe seven per cent are now covered, maybe even ten. But what about the others? And where are the bikinis for older ladies? Nowhere. What none of these brands have is a beautiful range of different kinds of bodies, reflecting reality. That's what body equality would look like. Not having to scroll through reams and reams of images of what, for most of us, is an unattainable body. I'm glad I'm nearly 40 and have some perspective on this issue and am no longer an impressionable teenager in the 95%.

The reaction to ASOS's frequent pushing of the boundaries always light up social media, I among many posted about their use of a non-airbrushed image in July last year as it was just so ground-breaking. Stretch marks! On a model. Reality? Whaaaaat?

What it shows us is that the world is ready for this change, even if Marketing Execs aren't. In the words of model Vivian for the Insider, 'It just highlights now more than ever that we want to see a wider representation of women and men on the high street and we are going to champion the brands that listen to us.'[115] I for one have a total shop-crush on ASOS and will be taking my business there as much as I can.

Postscript – in 2020 Rhianna's lingerie line SavageX would be a brand that would progress further towards what body equality in online shopping should look like. Still not on the homepage but in the main body of the shop, the constant juxtaposition of varied real bodies is a breath of fresh air. Kudos.

I've Still Got Questions
11th May 2018

I tweet Asda – their new summer ad campaign has just hit the TV. My response:

When reality doesn't imitate art @Georgeatasda what's up with your new ad? 'We are bold, confident, vibrant, strong'… No you are 'underweight, thin-washing, body-shaming, out-dated, unreal' Reality does not look like that. You prove it yourselves!

I attached a screen shot of the ad, alongside an office / behind the scenes photo they'd shared on twitter, depicting themselves to have… the natural diversity of bodies.

Postscript They didn't reply but a year later, almost to the day, I noted a new ad campaign, this time with a curve model involved and I took it as a win. We need more of this please. Just this morning (2021), one of my contacts, @realistically.body called out Seraphine Maternity for branding their post birth jeans as the 'tummy tuck' and within 24 hours the website has been changed. Call. Them. Out. You, me and us.

May 2018 - UKPSFW

Through my new friend at Bridge Models (a diverse modelling agency), I was invited to an event – the UK Plus Size Fashion Week.

Optimism: We should definitely go!

Ambition: This will do the trick. Everyone there will be in support of the petition! This could be the absolute game-changer we need.

Doubt: Do we really have time to shlep down to London for this?

Self-Preservation: (Glancing down at the To Do List) No, no we do not. We have to:

- Make flowers
- Find a dress
- Book treatments for the hen do
- Confirm numbers for hen do two – book limo
- Create a Mother's Day promotion at work
- Make a Mother's Day photo calendar for Mother
- Do the accounts
- Go to work
- Make more flowers
- Pick the kids up
- Find a backdrop

Besides anything I'm already going to London this month and I can't afford it again!

Excitement: The tickets are only £12! Oh come on, let's make a night of it!

Ambition: Twelve quid is actually nothing.

Self-Preservation: You do realise we're in London *next* weekend too right?

Doubt: You're over-doing it.

Excitement: But I mean this could be IT! You could contact the organiser, get them to announce your campaign!

Ambition: She's right. Remember, if this campaign doesn't fly… you need to know you did all you could, that's all I'm saying. If it flops and you hadn't gone…

Self-Preservation: Oh alright fine!

I grabbed my bestie by the hand, last minute, we jumped in the car and on a sunny weekend, made a thing of it.

When we arrived, at a Shoreditch warehouse, I suddenly felt really self-conscious. In a flip of circumstances, I was one of the slimmest in the room and felt that everyone was looking at me, judging me, wondering why I was there.

Doubt: Erm, this feels wrong. Everyone is looking at us.

Excitement: Did you bring your paranoia buddy, they are not.

Doubt: They are. We shouldn't be here.

Ambition: Why not?

Doubt: We're too thin.

Self-Preservation: We aren't. Let's shelve that idea, we've got work to do.

Excitement: Ooh prosecco!

In the days leading up to the event, I had tried to make contact with the organiser through Instagram messaging and email but achieved no traction. I had hoped in person it would be easier but she waved me away. Not put off I recognised a number of BoPo influencers and set about working the room, gave out cards and elevator pitches to just about everyone. We met a couple of lovely girls running Positively Perfect and I was introduced to the team at Be Real. This is an arm of the YMCA and is dedicated entirely to creating a positive body narrative. Any brand can align themselves with Be Real's pledge calling for: the responsible portrayal of body image by the advertising, fashion, media and music industries as well as other relevant organisations. I recognised a BoPo influencer who I followed on Insta, who was really interested in my petition / campaign and was keen to help me promote it. So many new contacts, I was pleased. I'd achieved some of what I'd set out to. I'd taken my bestie, we'd had a good night, finished off with Lebanese food in Shoreditch.

Sure enough the next day, one of the influencers centred my campaign on their twitter. It gave the petition a small boost. As I followed all my new contacts on Insta, my account fizzled with activity too (that's as opposed to 'blowing up').

Meeting with Media Smart

I squirm writing this – have been putting it off for so long. In the run up to this meeting, totally at the last minute – on the train journey there to be exact – I discovered something new. Body image doesn't feature in the diversity conversation. At all. Take for example, AMV BBDO - they are the biggest communications agency in the UK and have been for 20 years and they write (in 2018): 'Our vision is to build a diverse workforce and an inclusive work environment that promotes and supports our effort to do the best work of mainstream influence. To us diversity means a variety of difference among people relating to factors such as age, employee level, gender, marital status, national origin, physical/mental ability, race, religious beliefs, sexual orientation and thinking style.'[2] It is a detailed vision of what diversity should look like but not exhaustive. Although their policy listed the many ways they seek to establish inclusion: race, sex, sexual orientation, disabilities etc. it doesn't mention anywhere, the difference of body image / shape. It is my hope that body image will come to find its home under the diversity umbrella in the not-too-distant future. At the time I reflected that just like racial equality and sexual equality before it, body equality can become a darling of equal rights and not too soon either. I

[2] The AMV BBDO website has journeyed through changing the wording to their policy which much better encompassed inclusion. Now it has shifted again to a much simplified, one-page website (www.amvbbdo.com) where there is no reference to their diversity ethos and principles. It does however feature a new, beautifully diverse homepage to their website that speaks a thousand words.

thought it best to tweet senior management at AMV BBDO to highlight the issue and see if perhaps I could have a meeting with them while I was in London.

Their assistant replied via email that unfortunately the contact was out of the country but had recommended that I could meet with a connection at the Advertising Association who has done some great work on body image in ads. And it must have been some kind of serendipity because of course Media Smart is run by the Advertising Association and as I was about to discover, is in the same building, so I was already on my way! I set up a meeting, which ends up being a group affair with myself, the representative from the Advertising Association and the representative from Media Smart. And it's really heartening to see what is already being done. Media Smart has some incredible resources online to support teachers, youth group leaders and parents / carers. The Advertising Association show me they have developed a great magazine-style resource to address the issue of body image in high schools and youth groups. The only problem, with both is that they are trying to put over the content by way of the *usual fantasy body* format. Can they honestly not see it? Not modelling reality, visibility or body shape diversity at all.

And I ask what's next? The conversation went something like this…

Advertising Association: What do you mean what's next?

Me: I mean, the research shows that one input of learning around body image isn't really impactful against the flood of idealised messages we receive. And I'd say general awareness of your resources is pretty low. What's the next stage? Roll out? Curriculum change? Policy change?

The room cools.

Advertising Association: The UK Advertising industry is world-class! The fact that we are doing this *at all* is above and beyond any other country in the world.

Me: I'm not saying…

Advertising Association: What *exactly* are you doing here?

Me: Erm… I er, I've got this petition… I care about body image (should have said I'm writing a book but at the time I wasn't - in a rush I blurt out) I'm campaigning for greater body diversity in advertising. I want to know how we can improve things. What's happening behind the scenes, as it were.

Media Smart (clearly embarrassed): My colleague is very… efficient, can be direct.

The meeting ended soon after. Clearly I wasn't viewed as an ally here or had anything to offer. So just to be clear, these are initiatives paid for and developed – and developed well I should add, room for improvement but they are great resources – entirely by and at the cost of the advertising industry. The advertising industry recognises that it has a problem and rather than fix it, has created educative tools to show people, especially children how to please 'interpret' their skewed work.

Also, they keep calling it 'media literacy' – I suppose to infer, guiding people on how to 'read media', but I'd argue, it is more of a translating / de-coding experience. Has anybody heard of Media Smart? Around this time and since then I've asked many people, teachers, parents. And sadly, mostly no they haven't. You'd think for an advertising industry, they might have had a bit more success in raising awareness, pushing a campaign, you know, *advertising* it. Anyway I concluded the answer to 'What's next?' was… nothing. Box ticked.

I later discover that both the contact at AMV BBDO and the one at the Advertising Association are decorated by the queen. If you're wondering if I'm feeling out of my depth… you bet I do!

While I was in London, in a bid to drum up support, I also delivered letters (shlepped London) to the management of numerous celebrities as well as BBC Women's Hour, with a mini cactus each and a card with one of the body image stats on. I got no reply or support on social media. It's not what you know…

Postscript: In 2021, on Instagram, Media Smart has 505 followers. To put that into context, I have 1040; but I'm a sociologist, not an influencer… or the advertising industry. Media Smart was radio silent between July 2018 and January 2021 but is currently putting out some great content – albeit education around what is branded content, and piracy; not the skewed optics that we need to decode, but still worth a follow @mediasmartuk

May 2018

At Christmas each of us ambassadors received a Christmas card with our group picture on it and a bauble from Breast Cancer Now. Then in spring of 2018, something unexpected happened, I received a package through the post. Inside was a wooden box with a sliding lid reading M&S Summer Ball. Inside it was some foliage and an invitation to a corporate party raising awareness for breast cancer. How exciting! Our ambassador's Whatsapp group lit up as we started to prepare for the big event, we booked a nearby hotel, discussed our outfits and generally got rather excited.

The event was held at the waterside venue, Old Billingsgate in London. We arrived, the sun was shining, Tower Bridge was in our view, we posed for photos outside. We were greeted by two stilt-walkers in floor-length shimmering green curlicue dresses with flowing waves of hair, crowns of flowers and ivy and real blooms and bouquets around their dresses. The entrance also festooned with flowers and petals and inside, the ceiling hung with more foliage, flowers and twinkling lights.

We sat for dinner, the food was lovely and drinks were flowing. Better yet, Paloma and Kylie were performing! Both have had their own experiences with breast cancer and I knew that Paloma had done a soliloquy about body image at a local gig in Delamere. The night was incredible but all of that took second billing to the fact I had been seated next to the Director for Communications for M&S. As the evening unfolded, I told him about my work, about the blog I'd written about bikinis and where M&S sat within it, about my campaign, the petition. All of it. He listened, he was really engaged and motivated to learn more. I'd had cards made up with stats on them, which I showed him, I kept them in my purse. At the end of our meal and once the speeches had been done, he motioned into the crowd. As a man came towards us, I realised it was the man who had just given a speech and thanked us for our part in the campaign. It was the CEO of Marks and Spencer! We talked, he gave me his card and was also super engaged in what I was saying. A call then to another man, this time the Head of Marketing. I couldn't believe it. This was it! I'd got in front of the right people and they were listening! A meeting would be set up and I was to come back and present my work to the Head of Marketing.

Us ambassadors danced the night away, when Paloma sang *Make Your Own Kind of Music*, my co-ambassador and good friend Laura turned to me and said 'This is your song!'. We drank, we laughed, we couldn't believe where we were or how we'd got here and eventually found our way back to the hotel. Our association with

M&S is the gift that keeps on giving, not least in the friendship stakes too. I did not sleep a wink. I couldn't believe it, my body fizzed with possibility. I had no idea what this all meant but I was pretty sure it meant something.

Follow up email:

I wanted to say thank you for such a wonderful evening on Thursday, it was totally magical and I understand it raised a significant sum! Myself and the other Breast Cancer Now ambassadors had a wonderful time and it was so lovely for us to get back together again. We have a special bond.

I also wanted to say thank you for listening to my thoughts and making the necessary introductions. Over the last three years I have been compiling cutting-edge research available on the subject of body image and its relation to marketing. I am delighted that it might be useful and hope that it can contribute to raising the visibility of diversity.

I have now set up a meeting with your Marketing Department. It would be fantastic to be able to share the information wider too, as an industry-cultural-shift of this kind would need all departments on board.

I believe there are a number of 'stories' M&S could tell to ameliorate society's body perception, and serve your brand too.

Anyway, I won't keep you, just wanted to say, loved it. Every minute.

All best

Emi

And that's how I started working with brands as a Corporate Real Bodies Consultant, to help organisations to integrate the natural diversity of bodies and associated values into their culture, messaging and ethos. It's no use one person being enlightened, it has to be a culture-wide shift. It began with presentations and speaking engagements with senior staff at M&S throughout the following couple of years. It was heartening in Autumn 2019 to visit my local store and see the visual diversity that was starting to be injected in their lingerie branding. I liked to think I had a role in doing that and even though a tiny drop in the ocean, it meant that more women were seeing more of themselves represented in the world around them. So another little win for me.

22nd May 2018

During the campaign Amy Schumer's film *I Feel Pretty* came out. The premise is, a young woman takes a knock to the head, comes round and even though her body hasn't shifted at all, her brain believes she's gorgeous. It's a comment in how believing you are beautiful is very attractive. I liked it, of course. (I have since had it pointed out to me how messed up that premise is, that you have to have a brain injury to believe you're beautiful, also the concept of *Isn't It Romantic*. My bad)

I thought, this could definitely spring-board my campaign. I wrote a *My Real Life - I Feel Pretty Moment*, based on the mental shift that my cancer had brought me. I submitted to newspapers and magazines. I followed up with the *Female* section of the Daily Mail. My contact (a woman) responded:

This is not something the men in charge would want to run.

I am sorry what? I think someone just did a boob. The men? In charge of *Female*? I went on to call my contact back. I'm writing a blog, could you clarify what you said, I repeated it back to her. She quick-smart got off the phone to address it.

An email came through:

Dear Emi,

I am so sorry but I have just read through your piece again realise I have had my wires crossed. This is definitely something we would cover – as we have done many times before.
I'll give you a call in the morning anyhow and we can discuss further…

Didn't happen. No call, no published article, no support for the campaign. Nada.

Emi Age 39

I'll not resize this ring yet because…. you may lose weight before the wedding.

Emi Age 39

On ordering a chocolate mousse for dessert. 'Remember you've got a dress to fit into.'

Emi Age 39

A woman, stranger, at Croyde Bay, Devon, when I'm the only one in the sea not wearing a wetsuit. The sole comment of:
'Well the good news is, you'll lose weight that way.'

13th June 2018 - 800 signatures

Mike Amesbury
Labour MP for Weaver Vale
House of Commons

Dear Ms Howe

I hope you are well. Please find attached a copy of a letter I have received from the Minister for Women. As you will note from the letter there appears to be have been some crossover due to the shifting of personnel at government level.

I'm afraid this response is quite non-committal in terms of your specific goals, but instead goes on to outline what the government says are its wider commitments with regards to body image and the advertising industry.

With regards trying to secure more media attention for you, I'm sorry to say we have had no feedback this far despite approaching women's editors at newspapers and as well as the TV shows, all of which I was hoping would be interested in your story and goals.

There are members of my team with media background and they tell me that, unfortunately, the media is often 'trends driven' and moves in cycles. While one issue is deemed of value one minute, the next it isn't, then suddenly it is again.

With this in mind I will continue to keep my eye open for opportunities which I believe may be of use or interest you.

Please don't hesitate to contact me if I can be of any assistance on this or any other matter.

Yours sincerely,

Mike Amesbury
Labour MP for Weaver Vale

The Minister for Women's letter starts by re-directing the responsibility to the Department for Culture, Media and Sport, highlighting its links with the advertising industry. She tells me, there has been a recent consultation by the ASA on harmful gender stereotypes initiative. In fact she keeps talking about gender stereotypes and about trying to get rid of them 'once and for all' also that 'we have delivered an extensive programme of work on body image.' She mentions Media Smart as their pro-active action taken to improve understanding and resilience among young people. She also talks about frameworks suggested for teaching body image within PSHE lessons and 'recommended resources for schools'.

She mentions working alongside *This Girl Can*, and a number of further statistics relating to women's exercising habits, without addressing any of my concerns.

In short, I learn nothing new.

Wedding Day

Ours was an alternative wedding. Surprise! We got married in a glass house in the rose garden of our local park. In lieu of my Dad, our son danced me down the aisle, our daughter was Best Girl. The sun shone and marked the beginning of the heatwave of 2018. The dress code was vintage and the flowers were all paper. My hair was bright purple, as was my underskirt.

The day before, the Mums, Aunty Aileen, sisters and friends helped to decorate the two venues. Which included a rainbow ribbon backdrop and paper pom poms, streamers and garlands.

I had tried to do the whole, take your girls to choose the dress thing, and it just felt wrong. I couldn't justify spending that much money for a start. I think we went to only one wedding dress shop. The biggest barrier for me was the weight of the dresses. I wanted to feel free to move and dance, not dragged down by a dress.

In the end a friend sent me a link to one she'd seen (thanks Ali). I ordered it from Next online and tried it on, on my own, in a high street changing room. It was perfect, a strapless white tea dress with sheer shoulders and gems. My M&S cashmere jumper remains the most expensive item in my wardrobe!

And dance I did.

We had an ice cream bike, vintage street entertainers, a live band and a barbeque. Many people had changed into their slacks by dinner time. I spilt ice cream down my dress. In lieu of speeches I sang my HUSBAND a song, with my kids in the band.

We first danced with the kids. We sat round the campfire until the early hours. I felt free, and happy and didn't think about my body once. It was such a happy event! Thank you Universe!

Campaigning for Equality

A Reply to the Minister for Women

I received your letter, apologies for the late reply I have just returned from my honeymoon.

I was disappointed with the standard Media Smart quote you gave. Yours is the third letter I have now received from government quoting Media Smart as a catch-all solution to this problem. In reality, Media Smart is extremely underfunded, is an unknown entity and as such is not fit-for-purpose. I'd like to propose that we now need to take a more mindful, considered 'smarter' response.

I'd like us to consider what the existence of Media Smart reflects. Media Smart exists to try to offset the harmful coding and messaging of media and advertising.

Media Smart is packaged as 'Media Literacy'. This is a misnomer. Literacy relates to reading and writing, not decoding, translating and putting ideas, concepts and images through a 'reality filter'.

Not to undermine or in any way take away from the good work being done by Media Smart and the Advertising Association with limited means, however research finds, such initiatives to be largely ineffective in their objective.

'Several studies have found limited evidence of the effectiveness of media literacy, suggesting that the pervasiveness of the media's promotion of the thin-ideal is far greater than the pro-active messages offered in one-time interventions. Thus short-term media literacy interventions alone may not suffice to counteract massive media exposure to the thin ideal. Perhaps of greater benefit would be to reduce the emphasis on an unrealistically thin ideal that is perpetrated through the objectification of women's bodies in the media.'

(Grabe et al., 2008[116] – also Irving & Berel, 2001[117]; McVey & Davis, 2002[118]).

It is also apparent that the boards of the Advertising Standards Authority and the Committee of Advertising Practice are not guided by real-world representation, which might include: social commentators, healthcare workers, equality ambassadors but instead invested parties whose knowledge and experience are esoteric to the business.* I would argue this does not give them an impartial, broad, diverse view and that perhaps their attitudes are ingrained in the historical methodology of the advertising business.

I realise this may not be on your agenda, but as Secretary of State for Women, I feel that it should be, now and going forward. For too long now this issue keeps getting buried. But we can do better. My talks with the Advertising Association tell me that the existence of themselves and Media Smart, makes ours a 'World Class Advertising Industry'. But what of the social cost. Something which on asking the ASA, hasn't been researched, granted it is now under a, very quiet public consultation.

However being 'world class' is neither the same as being enough or adequate in the face of social and individual cost (please see research attached).

Can we make more progress on this please?

Yours sincerely,

Emi Howe

* In 2018 and at the time of writing, of the ASA Senior Management, ALL of the directors are white men, further, Senior

Management are entirely white and slim[119] Further: 'The Committee of Advertising Practice (CAP) and the Broadcast Committee of Advertising Practice (BCAP) are chaired by James Best, the Committees are made up of representatives of advertisers, agencies, media owners and other industry groups, all of which are committed to upholding the highest standards in non-broadcast and broadcast advertising.' [120]

This letter did not receive a reply.

Last ditch attempt – 5th July 2018

As a last-ditch attempt to go viral, before the petition closed, I organised a Thunderclap – this was a method of posting your message on the social media live feed of 100 people who agree and sign up. It has since become defunct due to shifts in social media functionality.

I post to Facebook:

We're over half-way with 54% of supporters needed for this thunderclap campaign in less than 12 hours. Can anyone else add their support. This is NOT the petition. Please take a look. It only takes 2 ticks. Ta x

I got 100 people to sign up. It did nothing, to the point of me wondering if it had even happened. It had though. If 100 people sharing a petition does nothing, what hope is there to go viral? I love that I got 100 people to help me though.

July 8th 2018

A week after I returned from our honeymoon, the petition closed with 968 signatories. Less then 10% of what we needed. 968 is still a lot, if you think of them in a march or, it would be impressive.

Ambition: Shall I update the socials?

Self-preservation: No

Frustration: Yes!

Self-preservation: What will it achieve?

Frustration: It will let them see, you did *all that work* for nothing! That *they* didn't do enough.

Optimism: Who's they?

Frustration: Them, everyone.

Self-preservation: And no one.

Doubt: No, *I* didn't do enough. I should never have taken this on *and* a wedding with young kids and another job. I should have left this for someone more able to devote more to it. And for a time when there's more awareness around the subject.

Self-preservation: There's nothing productive we can achieve by sharing how we're feeling now.

Excitement: Stupid.

Self-preservation: No! Depleted.

Doubt: Who am I anyway? '*What are you doing here*?' What did I think would happen?

Excitement: I'm *so* sorry.

Ambition: Maybe we could write a piece about it? Try one last time. Appeal?

All: No!

Frustration: You know the 'Make hedgehogs a protected species' petition has gained 21,000 signatures.

Self-preservation: Let's just give ourselves some time.

Postscript: I later discover hedgehogs are nearly extinct. So obviously still important. I was only jealous of the masterminds at hedgehog HQ.

The Gender Stereotype Public Consultation for the ASA

My response

I compiled a report of my findings, it was a 7000 word document! I have condensed it for you here. My main objective was to outline the clear risk to health and wellbeing that the current status quo creates. I have looked at the work of body image researchers Gemma López-Guimerà and Shelly Grabe, who conducted meta-analysis (the results of many studies) to draw their conclusions, amongst many others.

Is the research on the body image/media connection sufficient and reliable?

- Almost twenty years ago Stice and Shaw [121] identified more than a hundred studies where findings showed evidence that 'body image disturbance' informs and predicts eating disorders. Today the research on this subject is vast.

- 'Overall, many well controlled, randomised experiments have demonstrated an effect of the thin-ideal media on women's body image... the majority of evidence from these experiments indicated that brief exposure to the thin ideal body often leads to short-term adverse outcomes in women's body image and related concerns.' Grabe, 2008[122]

- What is the causal link, why is it a problem? It is a problem because, 'viewers begin to accept media portrayals as reality.' [123]

'A finding linking media exposure to disordered eating behaviours and beliefs should warrant public attention.'
Shelly Grabe, 2008[124]

Does the media impact on body image?

- 'A substantial portion of media content consumed by children is replete with unhealthy messages about the beauty ideal, body size, food, weight control and gender roles." (Greenberg et al 2009[125])'

- 'Adolescents are extremely influenced by external factors today. Such factors include, but are not limited to, family, religion, education, technology, and media. 'Among these, the mass media have been identified as the most pervasive and the most powerful.' (UK Essays, 2018[126])

- 'Evidence is accumulating that repeated exposure to media and to both the direct and indirect (via media's effect on peers, parents, physicians, etc.) pressure from media to be thin, constitutes a risk factor for body dissatisfaction, concerns overweight, and disordered eating behaviours in adolescent girls and young women.' (López-Guimerà et al., 2010).[127]

An impossible standard has been set.

- It's getting worse not better: '…we found that the effects were stronger in the 2000s compared with the 1990s.' (Grabe, 2008[128])

- 'It makes you feel disheartened. As if you're not going to be good enough until you're like anorexically thin' Age 15 from Devon, (Be Real, 2018)[129]

I finished my report with: What would Change look like?

- 'Interestingly, Dittmar and Howard (2004) found that women reported less body-focused anxiety after exposure to attractive, average-sized models than after exposure to no models; the lowered anxiety, in a sense, demonstrates a relief effect. Importantly for the advertising industry, research in this area has also demonstrated that when average-sized models and ultra-thin models are equally attractive, they are also perceived as equally effective in advertising a product.' (In Grabe et. al., 2008[130])
- Change would require a shift, 'a culture change across industry' (British Youth Council, 2017[131]). It would mean advertisers would need to get creative around how to sell products using a different format and narrative. Attitudes and norms would need to adjust as the public consciousness around this issue is raised.

Brands are already shifting

Brands are definitely already making moves in the right direction, however it is often piecemeal, the odd post on social media, it rarely translates to online listings or in-store branding (the exception being

ASOS who are leaders with online diversity). The shift, which really does only pay lip-service to the issue, indicates that it is incentivised by current trends rather than a responsibility to social health and wellbeing, or moral awareness and could easily shift again in the absence of minimum industry standards. What it does show is that a much-increased level of diversity is possible, is still sellable and useful in the world of sales and marketing.

And Another Thing

I also questioned CAP's confidence in being a self-regulating system. From CAP:

'By practicing self-regulation, the marketing community ensures the integrity of advertising, promotions and direct marketing.'[132]

This is specious logic and not one that is implemented in other industries throughout society – yeah, those folks are getting it seriously wrong, let's just leave them to it! No, there'd be investigations, reports, think tanks, revised legislation... In cases where constructs are harming wider society, self-regulation is not implemented as an adequate solution. From an onlooker's perspective, it is a rather convenient strategy for an industry which, historically has appeared very reluctant to tackle this issue. What's more, it seems to enable the industry's self-interest, especially in the face of claims that manipulations of an individual's insecurities is a driving force in advertising, as laid out in documentaries *Embrace* and *The Illusionists*.

To Conclude:

As in the case of smoking adverts of the past, the time is now to acknowledge the harmful effects of thin-ideal body image adverts, accept that even minimal exposure causes harm and more than 'self-regulation' is required id 'self-regulation' looks like this.

If CAP want to keep using their tag-line, 'legal, decent, honest and truthful'[133], and the ASA want 'Every UK ad to be a responsible ad', they need to consider how the values of support, inclusivity and compassion fit into their code and ask themselves why they aren't more demanding of their industry to better reflects those 'decent' values. If they really do care about 'unequal or harmful outcomes for adults and children'[134], CAP and ASA cannot ignore this issue any further.

I sent my report to: The ASA, M&S, to MP's Mike Amesbury (my MP), the Minister of State for Women, Minister of State for Digital and Creative Industries, Minister of State for Education and to the Royal Family.

The Aftermath

July 2018

Mike Amesbury

Labour MP for Weaver Vale

Dear Ms Howe,

Please find attached correspondence I have received from the Minster of State for the Department for Digital, Culture, Media & Sport in relation to your concerns surrounding body image.

Please do not hesitate to contact me if I can be of any assistance on this or any other matter.

Yours sincerely,

Within the letter is the Minister's acceptance that: 'The government recognises that pressure to achieve an idealised body image is a serious issue, … the recent Youth Select Committee Report, highlighted that increased time spent online (Emi: not the media then, the time) can lead to increased exposure to images of unattainable and unrealistic beauty.'

The letter continues: 'The Committee of Advertising Practice (CAP) has also just issued a consultation tackling harmful gender stereotypes.' The letter seems to indicate an assumption that many of my concerns would be addressed through this consultation. It implied that it will no longer be acceptable that idealised body images be portrayed as 'necessary for social or romantic success, or (in a way) which suggests young people should prioritise appearance at the expense of other qualities.' Which is what every advert has done, ever. Alright slight over-generalisation, but still! Adverts do this by linking positive outcomes - social, romantic or otherwise, to a narrow version of bodies. Remember affective conditioning - still doing that.

This statement vague as it is, suggests a lack of familiarity with the vast research I have outlined above linking media exposure (even a small amount) to negative health and social outcomes and the impact to mental health through normalising idealised bodies.

But there's more to come: 'More generally, the guidance makes clear that, while adverts "may feature idealised body shapes and physical features stereotypically associated with women and men (Emi: Ooooh so not changing anything), they should take care to avoid suggesting that an individual's happiness or emotional wellbeing should depend on conforming to an idealised gender-stereotypical body shape or physical features". What else would thin-washing all adverts say exactly? If pushed, do they mean that in an advert, they won't overtly say 'Hey, Seema, slim down so I can love you!' because they currently *do* imply 'Hey Patsy, slim down so you can be valid or visible in our society.' That's a pretty major social outcome right? I'm confused. Either way, it's now (2021) almost three years later and I haven't noticed any marked change. So I'm chalking that up to waffle.

British Youth Council

Youth Select Committee 2017 - A Body Confident Future

What the report *actually* said.

'Young people are more likely to be dissatisfied with their bodies if they are constantly surrounded by unrepresentative and unattainable ideals. The first part of this chapter considers what measures could be taken…

…the use of idealised body images in advertising is one of the factors which contributes to poor body image. In 2012 (Emi: 2012!) the APPG (All Party Parliamentary Group) on Body Image recommended that advertisers develop campaigns that more accurately reflect the diversity of the population. This was echoed by a number of our witnesses. For instance, Natasha Devon (Emi: MBE and fantastic advocate for body image and mental health) emphasised the need to use images of people 'of all shapes, sizes, ages and races' in advertising, so that 'the message we get is that there are lots of different ways to be attractive'.

The *Be Real Campaign* encourages organisations to sign up to their 'Body Image Pledge'. This involves using adverts which reflect the diversity of the UK; showing people as they are in real life (with alterations limited to technical corrections); promoting a healthy appearance; and promote the pledge. As Liam Preston, Senior Parliamentary and Policy Officer at the YMCA, and co-ordinator of the campaign told us:

'When you start to see people who look like you, who sound like you and who reflect your choices in life, that is when you start to feel more confident in yourself. So that for us was what we put front and centre of our body image pledge.'

Kate Dale and Liam Preston welcomed the support of brands in their campaigns. However, there is some concern that even those organisations who claim to be body positive are still perpetuating harmful norms. For instance *The Beauty Demands Network* (an academic-run multi-disciplinary network) suggested that, while advertisers may be using 'larger, fuller, fatter figures', this is 'often while conforming to other features of the contemporary beauty ideal.' In other words, brands may pay lip service to the idea of diversity but continue to emphasise the message that some conventional ideals of beauty are important.

The Committee welcomes the Advertising Standards Agency project in relation to harmful gender stereotypes, which we know can contribute to poor body image, and its commitment to formulate stricter rules in this respect. We agree that the rules on inappropriate sexualisation and adverts which suggest that it is acceptable to be unhealthily thin need clarification and look forward to the Committee of Advertising Practice bringing forward new rules which reflect this evidence by the end of the year (2017). However, regulation is only part of the answer – we also need to see a culture change across industry. This involves brands committing to using more diverse models and paying more than lip service to the commitment.' [135]

This report outlines everything I want to achieve, everything the research is pointing at and is not just about 'time spent online' but is, instead, clearly focused on advertising. It is also being, as far as I can tell, entirely ignored.

More Snazzy Envelopes

I'd got used to receiving thick envelopes emblazoned with the House of Commons' crest. This one had a royal emblem.

HRH 'receives a great many letters and requests from people associated with causes about which she cares passionately but, sadly, it would be simply impossible for her to respond positively on every occasion, no matter how worthy the cause.'
It was a kind letter.

A letter from The Department of Education – August 2018
'I am writing on behalf of the Secretary of State to thank you for your letter about the public consultation on gender stereotypes. Thank you for enclosing your response…

As schools are autonomous institutions, they are free to teach about media literacy and body image and may choose to do this as part of personal, social, health and economic (PSHE) education – a subject that can include a wide range of topics.'

Actually, not "As schools are autonomous"… rather "As we've not put this essential knowledge about the thing that we most rely on in the world, on the curriculum"… At least they replied!

Throughout this process I learn, not only will most politicians not answer the questions you ask them, but also there is so much shifting about of MPs in their roles, how are any of them meant to develop a specialty and the deep understanding of issues relevant to their subject if they're constantly brand new to the role? The current

Secretary of State for Education was Secretary of State for Defence last year.

Gender stereotypes in Advertising CAP and BCAP's Evaluation of Responses

The results are in and I get a reply! From this document I could see that alongside myself, others to comment were: The National Education Union, Girl Guiding, The Equality and Human Rights Commission. As an aside I do have a problem that this *public* document is written in legalese. I find it hard work. The response positions CAP as being in 'agreement' with everything they can, while using a lot of waffle. This in an attempt to hide their refusal to address the points raised – that's the basic message. As you'll see, the consultation respondents offer plenty of evidence to suggest that body image is *very* much a harmful issue, even a gender stereotypical one - if all girls are to believe they have to be thin and all boys strong.

CAP's direct response to my comments:[136]

'As noted in the consultation, CAP and BCAP consider that advertising is obviously not the only influence that can reinforce gender stereotypes, but the evidence indicates it does play a role. Their proposed new rule and guidance are intended to respond proportionately to the potential for harm that can arise from the depiction of these kinds of stereotypes in advertising. CAP and BCAP consider that the weight of evidence suggests that, while not all stereotypes are harmful or offensive, certain gender stereotypes can lead to mental, physical or social harm which can affect how people interact with each other and the way they perceive themselves wherever they appear.

CAP and BCAP note that advertising regulation in the UK works on the principle of imposing standards in order to prevent ads that harm, mislead or offend. The Codes do not impose quotas for inclusion in ads on the basis that this could infringe upon freedom of commercial expression.'[137]

Wow! They just came out and said it. Read that again! Or re-phrased:

Your inclusion doesn't matter as much as* our *money.

'CAP and BCAP consider that their proposed new rule and guidance are intended to respond proportionately to the potential for harm that can arise from the depiction of these kinds of stereotypes in advertising.'

Did they even read my research?

'CAP and BCAP note that the ASA has a strong position which prevents ads from depicting models in a way which makes them appear underweight or unhealthy, and from presenting an unhealthy body image as aspirational, as set out in multiple rulings.' (Then why is it still happening? Everywhere? The ideal body would be unhealthy for most people.)

'CAP and BCAP consider that the evidence around this issue indicates that the most significant potential for harm would arise from an ad suggesting that a person's happiness depends on conforming to an idealised gender-stereotypical body shape. This is reflected in the proposed guidance which states that an ad shouldn't imply that a person's body shape is a significant reason for being unsuccessful romantically or socially.'[138]

That's not enough. It is the norming of thin / idealised bodies. The flooding of messages that there's only one way to be, the use of affective conditioning, linking products to successful lives, certain outcomes that only look a certain way.

So, to round up, the ASA are committed to upholding complaints based only on models being 'unhealthily thin', and not outwardly shaming fat people. Can we have a round of applause please? For them succeeding to put in place the absolute bare minimum standard in response to this public consultation, or the Youth Council Report.

Meanwhile here's what the Girl Guides had to say:

- 89% think the ASA/CAP should publicly commit to making sure they represent all women fairly.

- 84% think they should commit to showing more positive female role models.

- 77% agree that they should agree not to show airbrushed images of women.

- 14% sometimes feel embarrassed about the way they look because they are not like the girls and women on TV.

- 37% of girls aged 11 to 21 feel they should try to look more like the pictures of girls and women they see in the media.

- Almost half of girls (45%) sometimes feel ashamed of the way they look because they are not like girls and women in the media. The numbers who feel this way increase from 36% among those aged 11 to 16, to 52% of girls aged 17 to 21.

39% aged 11 to 21 told us they often stop themselves taking part in fun activities because they are self-conscious about their appearance, and 30% take part less in the classroom/at work because they feel concerned about their appearance.

- 'Annoyed because it shows that women are only liked for their appearance.'

- Evidenced the need to tackle the common and unacceptable emphasis within advertising on women's appearances to the exclusion of their skills and abilities.

- Considers that advertisers should have a responsibility to consider the impact of their adverts on consumers' wellbeing. *(But what about their 'commercial expression'!)*

- Strongly agrees that the ASA should particularly consider the viewpoints of those represented in adverts (i.e. individuals watching adverts seeing their gender, ethnicity, disability etc. represented in adverts) over what is considered the 'general accepted standard' of what is offensive and acceptable. Considers it's important that individuals' views are considered over any such standard within society in that, as put by one of the contributors to

> the ASA report (p53), the society we live in remains 'institutionally and intrinsically sexist'.'[139]

And The National Education Union:

> 'Notes the APPG on Body Image heard evidence that girls as young as five were worrying about their size and appearance. Girlguiding research shows that 47% of girls aged 11-21 say the way they look stops them from doing everyday things they'd like to do and that from as young as seven, girls say they feel embarrassed and ashamed of how they look. Considers that challenging gender stereotypes is intrinsic for the promotion of positive body image. Believes this new guidance can play an important role in limiting the production of problematic and stereotypical ideas around body image for children and young people.'[140]

Here's the last I'm going to say on the subject of this consultation, while reading around the issue, I came across the 2017 document: *Depictions, Perceptions and Harm*, on the ASA website.[141] On page 37, I found these statements:

'This report assesses the evidence with the intention of isolating the role that advertising might play, if any, in contributing to harm associated with unequal outcomes for adults and children as a result of their gender…

It is evident that the overwhelming majority of research and grey literature on this topic is motivated by a reasonable concern to better understand the causes of real-world indisputable gender inequality – e.g. in relation to pay disparity and sexual violence. It is no surprise, therefore, that much of the evidence concludes that the status quo is not acceptable, and changes should be implemented to address evident inequality.'

Aside from the fact that negative body image effects are increasing over time, alongside our increasingly digital / unreal image-based worlds, this reads to me like, even if compelling research *is* presented, they aren't going to validate it, if it has been 'motivated' by anyone but… ah they're self-regulating… so anyone but them.

It also implies that such complaints are put forward by bumbling idiots who simply can't seem to grapple with 'real world inequalities'. That's how I read it anyway.

Moving On

For the rest of 2018 I threw myself back into my real job – body therapy – which I love and need like oxygen! But I always need a side hustle. The BABTAC industry awards were coming up and entry for Holistic Therapist of the Year included making a short video, which was the perfect distraction for me while I was licking my wounds. Everyone says I'm really good at my job, best treatment they've ever had, why not test the theory?

In January 2019 I got the news that I was a semi-finalist and would be traveling down to Gloucester to do a trade test. I was *so* prepped, I'd compiled a playlist, worked out my ultimate treatment sequence, convinced a friend to be my 'body'. It went well, I was happy, although unable to play my *incredible* playlist. After, we were asked questions. Then the examiner started asking me about my cancer - I'm always happy to talk about it, but it shifted the atmosphere a bit. I relaxed and chatted openly, she told me (as everyone does) about her friend or relative going through it. And then she hit me with one last question about aromatherapy oils and properties. I completely dropped the ball my mind blanked, why was I using grapefruit oil? I came back bumbling! Argh!

Close but no cigar. Looking back over recent years, I was used to disappointment. I know I felt… what's the point in my whole Bodequality efforts. I was tired. I couldn't see that it was ever going to change. It felt like it had all been a waste. So it was nice when…

Body Stories
Hannah

I received a WhatsApp from my sister-in-law. It's a tasteful naked photo! Below it is a caption.

'This is the first photo taken since I gave birth that I am happy with in terms of my body. Not because anything has changed. I can see all the things I don't like but my mentality has changed. I am swimming and looking after myself more but ultimately it's a mind switch. You can use this as you like, I just wanted you to know it's having an impact.'

To which I had a little eye-spill and replied:

'You're beautiful, gorgeous photo. Welled-up reading this, thanks for sharing it. There's so much opportunity for more joy and less pain to do with our bodies.'

Hannah replied, 'I know, it's quite incredible when you catch yourself after all the days when your body feels like it fails you but actually it's surviving and not only that, it's beautiful when you let it be.'

Hannah had also been the person to point out that, my work, out there in social media land, might not get loads of likes, comments, action, but is still making a difference. Making a difference to people that I will never know about. I treasure her encouragement – and her.

Husband got a little shock browsing our uploaded photos that night! Lols

Making the Most of 2019

June 2019 - An Email from The Telegraph

Hi,

I am speaking to various groups about the new ad rules on gender stereotypes which are being introduced on Friday. Is there anybody I can call from BodEquality to talk about this?
Just so you know, my news desk has asked me to ask people about particular adverts or common tropes in advertising that they hope may be stopped thanks to this new rule.

All the best,

We talked, I told him I couldn't offer a particular advert because the issue of body image concerns all adverts. By trying to pick out one, we're missing the issue.

This wasn't what he wanted to hear.

I followed up on email

Just an afterthought...
The fact we can't think of an advert that it would impact is a perfect example of the ASA and CAP's lack of agency. They seem reactive not proactive to social pressures/norms. I fully expect the same thing to happen regarding body equality. The hard work will be done by campaigners, lobbyists, brands going out on a limb, rather than any moral or ethical standards from them.

I've been told from the inside that we have a 'world-class advertising industry' but the best of a bad bunch does not make it good enough for the future I want for my kids.
Would be interested to read your piece.
All the best

Emi

Thanks Emi.
I fear the news editors will not run anything now, but hopefully I can get something in.

...They didn't.

With a bit of time two adverts do spring to mind that are in violation of this new ruling and are still on our screens. A chewing gum brand run an advert where two blokes by a water cooler are wearing the same outlandish shirt. One is short and fat and the advert implies that even though the fatter of the two, he gains approval through his choice of chewing gum.

A second advert by an insurance company depicts a Robocop style intervention after a robbery, only to arrive on-scene and be told the insurance company have already fixed it.

Robocop: I have to go... somewhere a crime is being committed.
Colleague: Er... Tom's been stealing out the fridge again.
Tom: No I haven't!
Robocop: Your move Tom
Cut To: Fat Tom running away.

2019 was peppered with attempts to create something out of all the knowledge and experience I had accrued. I spoke in schools, for The Women's Institute, Sister Hub - Chester's Women's Network, International Women's Day, at Chester Uni on Valentine's Day in a talk titled– *Falling in Love with Myself*, I hosted another screening with accompanying support pack, I created an evening event series called Body Nights[3], I'd even commissioned Amy to design the flyer; it sold no tickets. I now realise through pre-sales of this book, this might be a personal journey, not one people are comfortable doing in groups.

Eventually, I dragged my friends and contacts to a Think Tank evening around what a course on this subject could and should look like. I caught no breaks. Until, a friend recommended me for TEDx and I only went and got it!

[3] I now better understand, through pre-sales for this book, this is a personal conversation, a journey people want to take alone.

Inspiring Campaigners

I took the new train curve route into Liverpool to hear Gina Martin talk about her successful campaign to make up-skirting illegal, which she did. A man had taken a photo, up her skirt, at a festival and the police were powerless to help her. So she changed the law! I'd read her book *Be The Change: A Toolkit for the Activist in You.* Both the book and her talk were really interesting. It was heartening to hear about her own campaigning set-backs and frustrations. In her book she highlights the different ways you can petition and she looked at the drawbacks of using the official government petition website (which I did). From Gina's book:

'At the time of writing there are currently 31,731 petitions on the site, but only sixty have been debated (and, of course, it depends how you define 'debate'), and of the ten most successful campaigns of 2016, four were denied a debate and none have succeeded in their outcome or implemented real change. It's important to remember that if you're running a political campaign, at some stage you might want to hurry things along or put some friendly pressure on them, and that might be hard to do from their own petition site.'[142]

The upshot? I wish I'd used change.org, which also has improved functionality of sharing Facebook triggers etc.

Also, I'd like to take a moment to marvel at Gina's hutzpah - she's now still only 27 years old and has changed the frickin' law! She has achieved so much and is an icon of a generation that has all the power at their fingertips. And more power to them!

Promises Promises

For a long time I couldn't think about the campaign. I pretended it hadn't happened, I was embarrassed. I'm always putting myself out there and coming back empty. People must just think I'm a joke – that's what Doubt says anyway and he was on a bit of a one-emotion-mission during this time.

But time heals most things and it healed Doubt too. Then, and it's about time, something shifted and a veritable powerhouse of people lined up ready to come into my life. I have a client who takes a real interest in this work. He has a great breadth of knowledge on just about anything and we often see things in the same way. Our sessions were more like a career counselling session - I should have been paying him! Alan McKie - local Councillor and businessman. It was he who suggested connecting with my local MP back in 2018. He suggested I meet with local business-woman and recent award-winning Non-Executive Director, Dianne Walker. I knew Dianne already through serving on the Patient Participation Group for our local GP surgery and I knew she was super-savvy, I asked if we could meet. From the offset she was very supportive of my work so far and interested. She gave me a lot of great contacts, good advice and encouragement. Then, when Mental Health Awareness Day came around, bearing in mind in 2019, the Mental Health Foundation centred it around… Body Image (because it's such a massive problem), she put me in touch with a Manchester firm who were hosting an event. The company was called UKFast and they wanted me to come and do a talk, which of course I did. It was a great networking opportunity and afterwards I sent my UKFast, contact, an enquiry. I told her, I have all this knowledge and experience and I feel like it would work really well as a digital course. Perhaps I could monetise what I know?

They were also encouraging and let me know about a mentoring programme that they head up in association with Tech Manchester. The application date was coming up in June and they thought I should apply.

'Tech Manchester exists to provide start-ups with an opportunity to learn from those who have been there and done it, for projects to find the financial backing they need, and for the inquisitive to connect with like-minded innovators. Our goal is to lift Manchester's tech offering to new heights.' [143]

I went for it. It involved an application and if successful, which I was, I would be invited to a speed-meeting event. I would be matched with a number of potential mentors and get to pitch my idea to them. We'd then be best-matched and work together for a year to help get my idea off the ground.

That night, lying in bed with my husband… 'Listen I know, I've not made things easy for us. I'm aware that I'm in piles of debt for projects that I just can't leave alone. I know I could have just got a real job and we wouldn't be in this situation. Or even my actual job would be great if I'd just stop spending money on chasing wild geese!'

'But that wouldn't be you though.'

'Yes… Thank you. But this bothers me, a lot. I want to make a promise to you.'

'Right.'

I just need to put this into context for a minute. Recent to this, a colleague in his office had left to become a train driver, because the pay was much better.

'I need one more year. I want to promise you that if by June next year (2020), I haven't found a way to make a job out of what I know, I… will become a train driver… Why are you laughing!'

I don't know what's funny, I love driving, I'd make a *great* train driver! *Maybe* I still will!

'Right. OK' he was sort of bemused and as usual disbelieving. Honestly for fifteen years, this man has just kept coming along with me on ridiculous (costly) journeys that don't have a solid destination and have never got us a return. And he does it all for love! And he's fit. If by this point in the story you were starting to feel sorry for me, don't feel too bad; I won the husband lottery. He's literally the only thing that keeps me going sometimes. That and an incredible friend support network.

June 2019 - The Mentor Meet-Up

'I want to make online learning, for the corporate world, around body image. It's an area that needs attention and I have the tools to do it.'

Why?

- Because (insert any statistic) body image can have a massively detrimental effect on people's mental and physical health.
- Because unlike young people, the working generations have never been exposed to this kind of learning before. We weren't taught it at school. We can't reinforce our kids' learning, that we never had.
- Because it's a way to educate on a wide scale and raise social awareness.

- Because body shape equality deserves a place on the corporate inclusion stage beside every other inequality. It is not an acceptable discrimination.
- Because not learning this stuff is going to make people and by extension, businesses look like dinosaurs, when the kids get here!

Everyone was kind and interested but by far one mentor stood out to me. Atif Ahmed. He had the right energy: positive, upbeat, with a 'can do' approach. His day job is Head of Digital Product for BT, yep, he's The Business. We had to write down our preferred mentors and he was top of my list. Before the meeting ended, Atif caught up to me. 'There's someone I want you to meet.' Atif introduced me to Ivan, a film-maker. 'I thought you two were a really good fit.' I smiled and was polite but all I could think was, film-maker = money and I have none! Like… less than none. A lot less.

There was one other problem, Atif was the top of my list but he was top of someone else's list too. But before long, I found out that Atif had decided to take us both on as mentees for the year! BodEquality the specialist digital course provider on body image was born. It's tagline? Valuing Real Bodies. And Atif's other mentee? Ivan Moss, from Moss Creative later to be re-named Ivan the Great, because he is an astonishing film-maker!

First Mentor Meeting

My first meet with Atif, we met in a coffee shop in Media City. Atif has a great way of focussing my thoughts and vision, he has some brilliant ideas and suggestions and it was clear, this wouldn't be a quick fix of bringing my work to life. It was also clear, there would be no free or even cheap way to do it. Atif is easy to talk to and I was candid from the start.

'Atif, I've got something to tell you… If I don't make this work, I have to become… a train driver.' It's become a running joke - why does everyone find this so funny?

Atif kept my eye on what it would take to get my product to market. What are the steps, what can I do now, next, how can he help?

I did wonder what I was doing now in this 'tech' world. I have made a few websites in my time, using templates, for various businesses I've run but I knew nothing about online learning. I really had one big decision to make. Did I believe enough in what I was doing, to go further into debt for it?

Doubt: What the hell are we playing at? We've been here before.
Ambition: This is different!
Frustration: Different how? Impulsive idea, shoehorn everything into it, watch it flop.
Self-preservation: You might have a point.
Optimism: Have you lot literally got no vision? I can see how this plays out… Yes! The reason nothing has worked so far, is to keep her driven and motivated to achieve something more important.
Excitement: Yes! Totally, with no success whatsoever on the way #motivation #GoEmi!
Doubt: You do know that is the definition of insanity! Doing the same thing over and over again and expecting different results.
Ambition: Yes but this time, it could be different. We've changed.
Self-Preservation: I feel totally on the fence here.
Optimism: Ok forget about the debt, forget about everything. We're ninety, talking to our grandkids about our life. What do we say. We got here and then opted for a mediocre life, not one built

on our true beliefs and passions? Answer me this, if we don't do this, what will we tell them?

Doubt: Why do we need to tell them anything, just give them biscuits! They won't care.

Ambition: I suppose you're right.

Excitement: When you put it like that…

I made a call. 'Hi, is that Ivan?'

FHT Conference

I thought I'd have another crack at Therapist of the Year, this time with the Federation of Holistic Therapists. I'd entered these awards unsuccessfully in a previous year and this time I was a finalist. I headed down to London to the annual conference and ceremony.

During the conference, the FHT was also centring body image (because… it's really important) and I was of course interested to hear more about it. The speaker was Dr Fiona Holland, Senior Lecturer in Psychology at the University of Derby. Her special interests include: behaviour change, self-esteem, breast cancer and body image. I really enjoyed her speech which was all about how our industry can pivot in response to issues around body image. The wording that we use on our advertising, the damaging effect of 'fat talk', about body appreciation and how our role might fit into that.

I was able to briefly catch Fiona after her presentation and explained what I was hoping to achieve with BodEquality. She was very interested and we swapped details with a view to following it up later.

Third time unlucky, still no award but I felt that I was meant to be there to meet Fiona and I didn't feel like I came away with nothing.

November 2019

I reached out again to Caryn Franklin, presenter of The Clothes Show, former co-editor of i-D magazine and long-time fashion commentator, knowing she was a supporter of my campaign back in 2018 - I wondered if she'd be willing to feature in the upcoming course. She agreed that we could have a quick chat on the phone, during which she told me about an event she would be at, in the coming week and I should come along. It was run by The Fashion Roundtable and the event was called, *Are You Represented?* This was another rare opportunity of being in the same room as the right people. I already had more Autumn plans to visit London and, childcare aside, the credit card couldn't really handle *them.* Still, I juiced it up again, bought a train ticket, a hotel room, pulled up my big girl socks and set off for Shoreditch.

It was a really illuminating evening and I suspect now, somewhat of a rare opportunity to hear Caryn speak. A really diverse panel had been invited and it made for thought-provoking listening. Afterwards, I caught up with Caryn and asked her for some time. I asked her what the sticking points were with the status quo, why is the fashion world like this? So resistant to inclusivity.

Following the event, Caryn sent me this quote:

'The reason businesses are slow to move on the issue of diversity and representation is simply that most management teams are not diverse or inclusive in the first place and so the issues are relegated to a superficial conversation of 'diversity,' and something that has to be addressed tick-box style. Such mindsets will always view success through the lens of the quarterly profit return and shareholder endorsement. This means there is a strict adherence to reduced outgoings, not an expansive spend for marketing to promote a variety of body types, skin tones and ages. There is a lot of fear in the industry, that a step in any direction might negatively impact their profit margins.

A fashion shoot featuring a diverse concept does cost more money, simply by nature of the number of models used to portray difference and the casting days it takes to find the right mix of people. Plus sampling in a range of sizes ahead of production is an additional cost. And then there are fittings as extra when you are working with bodies that are not standard sizes. These are just some of the issues that deter management from embracing new thinking. I have experienced this short-sighted approach when everything is boiled down to costs on a balance sheet but it is a hard one to tackle. The numbers on the page are always prioritised. Yet presenting a range of diverse faces and bodies to the audience can impact on consumer sensibilities and significantly effect 'intentions,' to purchase and studies to show this happens. It's an unknown step for most brands to contemplate, especially in the current climate of retail insecurity.

As a founder member of All Walks Beyond the Catwalk, we called for imagery that portrays a broader range of body and beauty ideals. We began educational work to encourage enlightened thinking and empower young creatives to make the shift in not just physical representation but also in mindsets by embracing of emotionally considerate practice. Fashion has the powerful potential to shape personal identity and self-esteem, through its messaging. Our education programme encouraged developing fashion students to start from a diverse viewpoint and value its business potential and creative possibilities, not see it as an obstacle to success or profit. The reality is, consumer needs are not being answered or represented.'

www.franklinonfashion.com, **www.allwalks.org**

After the event, I walked back to my cheap hotel room in the rain but felt a sense that the night too would be significant.

Some of Caryn's points are echoed by Rita Clifton in her book Love Your Imposter: 'It's all very well to say that a business is only responsible to shareholders, but this becomes a proxy for making as much short-term profit as possible. The longer-term responsibilities of business – to generate sustainable wealth that employs people reliably and looks after customers – are as fundamentally important. It's also worth remembering that shareholders themselves aren't just faceless institutions. They're staff, pensioners, ordinary people with savings and a stake in society. And if we don't have clean air to breathe, if there are no resources left and the majority lead miserable lives, who cares what the quarterly results say?'[144]

Diet-Culture Gate

A flappy diet club banner materialised outside my kid's school. I was fuming! I spoke about it to some colleagues and contacts who knew the local diet club contact - she's a lovely lady. To me it was sad proof that so many people still have no idea how we're thin-messaging our kids, ourselves. So many people don't get that not everyone wants to be thin, can be thin, needs to be thin, nor relish the pressure on themselves, their kids. I spoke to our headmaster about it but it was next to, not on school property. I got the local rep's number online and made the call. My voice was shaking because who loves conflict? But also, I am so passionate about this. I asked her to take it down. She seemed a bit confused at first so I explained my work and background. She agreed to move it and suggested the park. I still wasn't happy. I didn't want it anywhere near my children or their route to school. It was a totally awkward conversation but it was successful. In the end the banner appeared on the outskirts of the village but much less obtrusive.

January 2020

My plans had all converged and the BodEquality Body Image Course was now becoming a reality. The reason I was keen to create content for this market is two-fold. Firstly, people of my generation, if they want this knowledge, have to go and find it and we largely don't. We weren't taught any of this in school so to me it seemed the best way to reach the largest number of my generation and above. Secondly, it's no use our kids getting this learning if they're bringing it home and not having it reinforced there. If their parents aren't genned up, how easy is it going to be for them to assimilate their new information? Day one of filming began in Cheshire. I had spent the intervening months, compiling lists of people I knew who I wanted to speak on my online course. Thanks to the 2018 campaign and all of my experiences, that list was long. I wanted to represent all kinds of people and their experience around their relationship with their body. I asked some clients and some people just randomly floated into my life. In the end I lined up 21 speakers, including Dr Fiona Holland, who I'd met back at the FHT awards. You see! I'd also brought together a script and pre-interviewed each person to compile what questions I wanted to bring out for each of them. I felt that each demographic was covered: gender, age, race, ability, LGTBQ.

We started Day One filming with me doing some pieces to camera. Ivan is eternally patient and encouraged me without making me feel daft. 'You've got to really over-egg it! Put loads of energy into it and smile! It'll feel too much but it will look and sound great!'

I trusted him and he was right. We started working well as a team, understanding how I needed to rehearse in order to get it right. There was take after take after take and I started to figure out what wouldn't work. A slight shift in my tone, a dropped smile at the last minute. On top of which we also filmed the speakers. But thanks Ivan, we worked so late that night!

Our next shoot was in London as that's where a lot of the speakers were. I hired a conference room in the Marriot Hotel, Maida Vale. I travelled down with Ivan and I'll admit I was apprehensive about the journey – bet he was too. Three hours is a long time to spend when you barely know someone! I shouldn't have worried though. We just chatted all the way, laughed, shared our life stories. Stopped for noodles. By the time we got back, we were firm friends! I learned a lot about him and I learned I was wrong. I shouldn't have just seen money when I met him. I learned he cares about the types of projects he takes on and he'll find a way and a budget to make it work, if it's something he's passionate about. I also know him well enough that I didn't mind asking him to find a way that I can pay him using a credit card! And I didn't mind paying because his work is worth every penny! We had one final day of filming, back up in Cheshire - February 2020. What followed is both the best and worst thing that could have happened.

How Covid Felt Like Cancer

I think my lasting feeling of this period in my life is unsettled. Feeling: Am I in danger? What does the future look like? This could be a catalyst to so many good things. Isolated and lonely. Time to think and feel and heal but on a grand scale. And like a roller-coaster. All very familiar feelings to me.

I remember during my cancer recovery thinking, I wish everyone could have a wake-up call like this, only without the pain, because for me it was the very best catalyst to change and finding my true path. Unfortunately, the threat is still here, but widespread awakening, I hope is underway. I hope enlightened minds come out of this.

Locked down from my day job, with dozens of film takes to sift through and kids just old enough to commandeer their own home-schooling, I'm not sure the course would ever otherwise have been completed. I spent hours, days, sifting through them all, making time codes, picking out soundbites, logging them on a spreadsheet, arranging them, editing them. I then sent it all back to Ivan.

One by one, the course modules in their rough form started to come through. What a rush! It was so exciting to see it start to take shape. The second edit was about sourcing images to complement the work. I was doing all I could at my end to keep it within budget (what budget? I don't know). I'd send the new files back to Ivan and once again he'd work his magic. I can't tell you what a thrill it is to see my ideas take form, for other people to do their bit and it become a tangible thing. Just the best high! The same goes for Amy when she sends through designs I've commissioned. Amy was also involved in helping to create animation parts of the course, with Ivan, we sourced voice-overs too. It was hard work, and seemingly never-ending. The kids, home-schooling did a great job and were largely self-sufficient. The sunshine kept calling me from outside.

And then we had a largely finished product. I'd put a 90-day invoice structure in place for those who needed paying, thinking that would be plenty of time to sell a course and offset the cost. Not in this climate sunshine! More invoices haemorrhaging my credit card. But we can't stop here pally! The website I was designing just wasn't working for what I needed, so I set about starting it from scratch on another platform. I had also put the work in and learned an awful lot about learning platforms, digital education portals, I'd networked my socks off and taken part in many, many, many, unpaid zoom events or podcasts. Looking back now, it's been so much work!

My next job was to try and figure out how to make it accessible for some early market research. I had a number of people who were willing to review the course for me and feed back. It took some time but eventually I had some helpful and encouraging responses.

Then I received an email from Caryn Franklin. Caryn was happy to sign off the quote she'd done for us, as long as the work contained both race and, if possible, faith diversity. She didn't want to be involved personally as she wanted, rather to make space for other voices who haven't had the opportunity of exposure that her privilege has afforded her.

I replied: 'I don't have an enormous budget but what I do have I am using to include a broad-spectrum diversity as it's really important to me too and hopefully an aspect we can further develop as the course grows in future reincarnations.'

I sent Caryn an early version of the course, excited to get her approval. She responded:

'The first illustrations are exclusively white. I'm glad the ensuing images are of a variety of skin-tones however, hairstyles are exclusively Caucasian and clothing is westernised with no faith representation.

These things are small if we can see ourselves but they are bigger if we cannot. Further they act as examples of unconscious bias – the thing you wish to challenge in others.

HR departments and individuals may feel challenged by non-inclusive imagery.'

It implied racism on some level in my content. I couldn't understand it, I'd gone out of my way to create a product that centred black people and a quarter of our speakers were from diverse ethnic backgrounds. When I followed up for clarification, Caryn explained it was in the silhouettes I used on my branding. The BodEquality branding is a colourful mix of lots of different body shapes and that is where I had focussed my mind - shape. On reflection I could see, they could all be interpreted as Caucasian. I was gutted, I just hadn't seen it. I live in rural Cheshire, I have black friends locally but on reflection all of their silhouettes generally could be construed as white. Look at my excuses! Thankfully we still had time to change it. Caryn gave me my first lesson on unconscious racial bias. I hadn't seen it because it is a problem that doesn't affect me. Mortifying.

How Covid Exposed Our Body Obsession

A Blog April 2020

Covid: the gift that keeps on giving… What did people do during the bubonic plague without memes? Without ways of connecting with others at distance about how we're feeling through a funny, catchy, heartfelt lens into other people's lives. The shared, isolated experience.

For the most part they're harmless and fun but there is one particular meme theme that I'm uneasy about. The *We're all going to be soooooo fat when this is over* meme.

These seem, on the face of it, perhaps an absolutely fine and fun way to communicate a shared concern. It's also a very British form of self-deprecating humour:

- 'Us after lockdown / quarantine has ended' – image: two jaguars puffed up like puffer fish.
- 'Wonder Woman after lockdown' – A before and after picture using the real Wonder Woman and a fat woman badly dressed up to look like her. An actual woman – she's out there somewhere.
- 'Meeting up with the girls after lockdown' – three fat woman fall out of a car
- 'Some time in the future – "well that's lockdown finished with, how do we get out la?" A fat couple portrayed as wider than their door.

I should also say that these have come from my social media, people known to me - good, kind people, not intended to hurt in any way. I take no relish in making the point, but it is something that we need to start having conversations about.

During the filming of the upcoming Body Image Awareness course, I was joined on-screen by people from all walks of life including Dr Fiona Holland. Fiona talked me through how 'fat talk' (talking about our bodies and weight / size etc) can have some really poor results on both our mental and physical health. Increasing depression, lowering self-esteem and self-regard. This is backed up by the research from the Mental Health Foundation which shows that feeling bad about our bodies is a marker for increased stress, and incidence of self-harm and even suicide. What the research shows is that these effects happen whether you are directly fat talking or if you are just over-hearing / seeing it. Maybe you can and maybe you can't relate to this. Either way, cutting back on communal fat talk might be a really healthy thing you can do, for yourself, your friends, your kids...

However further... in the gentlest, most supportive way I can say this (because I know it's just a lack of awareness, not intended to be cruel)... it's not just about you. Some people are not putting on weight during lockdown. Some people are maintaining or slipping back into their eating disorder restriction patterns or guilt exercising on account of the stress and lack of control. The memes for them could provide a trigger. We also need to remember, some people *already* look like this. It reminds them to feel (fat) shame about their bodies. Even though their bodies may be a result of trauma, accident, disability, hormone imbalance or an eating disorder. While we're on it, *this* year's Mental Health Awareness theme is kindness. We are absorbing fantastic messages during this challenging time to #bekind. This isn't that.

It creates unnecessary stress. For me, right now, food is providing me with the light and shade I'm sorely missing from the rest of my life. I'm choosing things from the supermarket I wouldn't normally buy. It would be really helpful if that small luxury wasn't tinged with negativity and was just a source of pleasure.

On a wider scale, normalising messages like these are the reason no one plays with the fat kid at school. Kids absorb messages around bodies... from us. Every fat talk comment we might throwaway, forms realities in young minds. The statistic that 81% of ten-year-old girls are afraid of being fat, is one that I can't shake. What are we doing, socially to give kids this message? We are obsessed with bodies! We keep *talking* about bodies!

During our talks, Dr Fiona Holland pointed out that our social media feeds are unrepresentative of our lives, leaning much more in the favour of posts about bodies and food as opposed to other parts of our lives or interests. This can also be seen amplified during this Covid period. There aren't a plethora of posts clean-shaming our homes or cars or gardens. Even posts about helpful things like books or TV series that people are enjoying aren't as apparent as the focus we're seeing on bodies and food.

As I'm editing this piece, the presenter has just asked a caller on the radio 'Are you putting on loads of weight during this lockdown?'

This is a really multi-layered subject and no one needs feel any shame. We have been sold a really simplistic view of superficial health. We can't know what we don't know. It's an awareness thing - hence body image awareness (or body intelligence) is a subject we can aspire to learn. This is not a message we have regularly received from the world around us. We have actually heavily received the opposite message in the name of commercialism, but you have to admit, it does make sense... to stop fat talking. This used to be a marginalised conversation, thought only to affect those on the periphery of society. And it's easy to make that mistake because it's an invisible problem, that we don't talk about. But it is a widespread, personal problem, an intelligent conversation, a thoughtful, forward-thinking one. Most importantly it is right. We need to change, if we actually care about our health and the health of others.

I was starting to form a strong idea and my work was consolidating. I shared this blog – still available at www.bodequality.com widely on my socials. You know what, no one commented, but I stopped seeing those memes

25th May 2020

Black Lives Matter

The death of George Floyd and the 2020 Black Lives Matters Movement hit many people like a blow. A trauma, to a captive, at-home audience. Despite my passion for equality and drive to understand, I kept failing. My first mistake was to hashtag #alllivesmater. Quickly I was corrected. This wasn't a stage for all lives - #blacklivesmatter. My instinct was sorrow, regret, remorse. Quickly I was told those emotions aren't welcome in this conversation. They aren't helpful and why should black people be the comforter in these circumstances, they don't want to have to make *us* feel better or deal with our sticky emotions. They also don't want to have to explain this to us. It has already been a labour they have had to undertake for a lifetime – to try and make people understand. To enlighten and guide the average white person into their world and argue over the injustices, of lifetimes. I put up a black square on my social media and quickly I was corrected. These black squares were flooding out black voices. I grappled with the messages, trying hard to get it right. Genuinely wanting progress. I can see how perhaps some white people may have got to this point of feeling failure and lost motivation or interest to engage. I learned that the only right thing I could do, was sit in that discomfort. And learn. I bought books, downloaded books, listened to podcasts, followed new people on social media and tried to take it all in, with an open mind. I saw my TV screen flood with black faces and black voices, every advert had black representation and part of me was so happy, this really did look like change, progress. But later black voices were hacked off at being tokenised and commodified. Did it feel a bit like being pushed stumbling onto a brightly lit stage, used for 'the optics'.

Out of everything I've written I am most nervous about writing this. So deep in it we still are and emotions so raw. As a creator, I was sure I wanted representation in my project and I sought out those people who could do that. It wasn't an organic process, but it came from a genuine place of wanting to represent reality – which as you know I care about a great deal. In doing so had I tokenised them? But not doing it would mean not representing them, which for me, would be worse.

I did what every white creator of content did. Got in touch with my black collaborators and asked them to create more content with me. I didn't get a response. I had very little money to offer now but I was concerned because throughout the course, had we really discussed race to the extent that it should have been? Especially in relation to body image - even with some slightly leading questions. I had wrongly assumed it was because things these days are much improved. People know how to be inclusive and what could potentially offend don't they? But in retrospect, I am a white women, the black participants may have felt wary of being *perceived* as 'playing the race card'. Or assumed it wasn't something I would want to centre. Or just have learnt to have a heightened radar for potential race-related awkwardness and steered well clear. Similarly, I was nervous of saying anything that might offend or get wrong. Regardless of why, I wanted so much to rectify that.

Of course *every* creator got in touch with their black collaborators and the feeling must have been overwhelming, with maybe a side-helping of incredulity. At the same time, situations which black people have had to normalise (white privilege, micro-aggressions, unconscious bias and overt racism) had surfaced and been validated as unacceptable. It must have brought up a lot of buried pain, trauma. I think the response, mine included, was fairly clumsy.

In my experience many white people will identify with not being racist without having given it much personal thought or attention. Like it's a status, not awareness. We need to be having difficult conversations. Like in the case of my course, conversations can be stunted because people are trying very hard not to offend or be offended and so instead no conversation exists. Do we need to hold space for that mutual discomfort, and be brave?

I'd also noticed something else. Support for the 2020 Black Lives Matters Movement was largely being created on social media by my women friends. I didn't see any of my white, male (in real life) friends engage with it. There is one male friend in particular who is vocal about just about everything and anything. He is eternally inquisitive and prepared to ask questions. Especially if it's political and he had been conspicuously quiet. Todd is a friend of mine from my high school days in the Midlands and now runs Spaghetti Besties - digital marketing advice in a Facebook networking group. I kept watching the socials to see if he would make a move and then he did. Reproduced with his permission:

Facebook - Todd - Spaghetti Besties - 12 June 2020

Real talk...

Is racism a big issue in the world YOU'RE in (not the media world). I don't see it in my day-to-day life at all, but that's my narrow focus. As a white man (apparently that's what I am, I don't see myself as a colour) I don't see it as a massive issue, but is that wrong? Am I in a bubble? Am I so 'privileged' that I don't see the problem in front of me?

We're all different. I get that. We have choices. We choose what we believe and who we trust.

I'm also very onboard with the notion that we all judge each other because it's a part of our inbuilt autopilot to protect us.
I don't see that as a bad thing, it's just natural. To carry on thinking bad of folk because of appearance is a choice, an uneducated one in my opinion.
So... is it really as bad as this whole shit storm is making out? I honestly never knew it was this bad... here... in the UK.
I live in Warwick now, but I was born in S.E. London which had everything ethnicity represented and my best mate at school (Chun) was Chinese.
I don't remember it being an issue at all. My grandparents were racist. That was 'normal' for them, but neither me nor my brothers really bought in to it. I hope we didn't, anyway.
I dunno... I just don't see it as an issue but I'm worried I've been rather naive.
You guys are a sensible lot and I expect a sensible debate here.
The post received 358 Comments…

It was really fascinating watching, in one day, a white privileged man, change. And this is an important demographic, I think because this demographic has less (or sometimes no) experience of discrimination, the colour blindness is real - the inequality blindness too! They are the straight and true trees in the middle of the forest. He was gently corrected, he was also humbly prepared to be wrong and held space for the discomfort. If you're wondering what this section has to do with my work, it's this. Skin colour is an important part of body image and self-image but further, for those who are fat and black – or fat and queer, fat and disabled… the struggle, the disconnection, the experience is amplified. Secondly and vitally, there is a lot in how he did it, that we can learn from, replicated in others to better understand the BLM Movement and can be applied to other forms of perceived invisible inequality – like fat-shaming for example. I want to show how Todd dealt with it because he was beautifully non-defensive about it. Those who don't live with prejudice, most likely are not aware of it, might just lack experience and yet I know it's hard to be wrong and a man in this world. There is too much blinkered vision where: *the world feels right to me and I feel safe in it, why would I discomfort myself with someone else's view.* However that discomfort is a signal of the privilege of our everyday comfort around our bodies.

Here are some of the replies to Todd's post:

Comment: Not seeing colour is a huge problem because it denies and negates other people's experiences. The USA, UK and much of the world is set up to systemically favour and benefit white people and to oppress black people and people of colour. Please watch 13th to start to learn more.

Todd: I see it! As in I know my friends have grandparents from other countries. I just don't see that as a problem.

Comment: And that's the problem. It IS a problem for them, therefore for all of society. Listen to voices that are not having a white experience.

Todd: Ok x

Comment: This is white privilege. People of colour have a different experience with daily micro aggressions that they usually don't fight because it's too exhausting. If we are to redress the balance, we all need to educate ourselves. Thanks Todd for raising this. I love that you are willing to explore.

Comment: Please can I encourage you to read this post by my friend Kerrie (reproduced here later). I think it's a helpful (and difficult) insight into the world of everyday racism in Britain for those of us lucky enough to have not really seen it for ourselves xx

Todd: (after reading Kerrie's post) That's made me so sad. What world are we in?

Comment: Do we not think it's down to our experiences and perception and therefore our sensitivities? For example as a tall, blonde woman I have been subjected to sexual harassment and discrimination over and over again. In fact I'd say that at most networking events I attend, I get at least one man making a sexist comment or asking me about 'my kids and husband' (I have neither and think it's irrelevant). So I am 'sensitive' to that and will identify it quickly and just ignore it in most cases. It's only recently that women were suppressed, couldn't vote and were considered the property of their father or husband ... well past the abolishment of slavery. And we're still fighting for equality in business today.

Todd: Thank you. This actually makes more sense and I can understand this and map it out into race. I guess on some level we all experience 'conditioned' behaviour and as a white man in the UK, I'm unlikely to have ever had that.

Comment: You might not feel privileged but if you had different colour skin you'd have had to work harder for the same success and recognition. It's that privilege we have to accept we've benefited from in order to change it.

Todd: That's a good point and one I'm looking into.

Comment: It's a far deeper and bigger problem than most people realise and it's harder to see when you're not affected. Also people don't want to see it. Because it's very uncomfortable viewing.

Todd: Agree. I wanna see it tho. I don't want to be blind to this.

Comment: For me the ownership or racial stereotype jokes is the key - I will happily joke but if someone else does it....

Todd: Shit, yes, I do that to you. F*(k. I need to re-evaluate some stuff

Gus Bhandal (BodEquality contributor): Oh mate, where do we start?

How about the number of times I was attacked after 9/11?

Or being told after Brexit: 'You're next mate'.

Or the POTUS building a wall to keep Mexicans out?

Or our own PM calling Muslim women 'letterboxes' (plus much more).

And that's just the serious stuff.

Even recently, someone thanked me for coming to their networking group by saying they 'welcome diversity'.

Or how about the woman who came up at another networking event to tell me all about her recent trip to India… and then walked off.

Or people asking 'what curry do you recommend?'.

Thankfully, much of what I hear is born out of ignorance and lack of learning, as opposed to nastiness.

And I love answering questions – whether about India, or turbans, or anything that helps someone else understand more about me and my culture.

Banning Fawlty Towers or Little Britain, or Keith Lemon apologising for his *Bo Selecta* characters, is just stupid. I love a good bit of racial stereotyping, because the joke is supposed to highlight the stupidity of it.

I think concentrating on most of this stuff just trivialises the actual, genuine, pure evil racism that many people of all colours and races, encounter on a daily basis.

As a British Indian, the biggest irony is that I'm seen as an outsider in both Britain AND India, which kinda makes me homeless.

However, weirdly, I'm one of the lucky ones. The stuff I've encountered as a brown guy pales in comparison to what some people go through on a daily basis, but I can only tell you about my own experiences, obvs.

So to answer your question, it raises a thousand more questions. Racism is everywhere but it's very easy to miss. There are varying degrees of racism and it's not as simple as… er… black and white.

Todd: Look at us all taking about a deeply emotive subject and not shouting at each other, but instead listening and learning. This is such a brilliant and uplifting result of a post I genuinely was nervous about putting out there.
Comment: YouTube: Privilege/Class/Social Inequalities Explained in a $100 Race - Please Watch to the End. Thanks.
Todd: Holy crap. That's incredible. Thank you. Thank you so much for sharing x
Todd's partner: I sent this to you a little while ago but I don't think you were ready for it then.
Todd: Sorry. I don't think I was.
Todd's partner: If you were truly racist I couldn't be with you. You're just not anti-racist – which is what you're aiming towards.

I reached out to Gus via email for further guidance on this chapter. His reply:

Hi Emi
Todd's group is full of sane people. Go look at football or Formula One pages, and see the absolute idiots that hang out there, because they don't like Lewis Hamilton for being black or 'boo' when players 'take the knee' before matches.
It's a VERY deep issue, one which we will never put to bed - but the main thing is that you are tackling it and offering opinion and thought, which is just as important as anyone else's, and that is more than can be said for most people.
If you need anything else, or a follow up chat, etc, please do shout - always happy to help.
Gus x

Like any big change or shift, the pendulum is still swinging. We are still in the limen - we have yet to settle into *another* new normal, which will hopefully be greater awareness and a racial equality many levels above where we were pre-May 2020.

I want to take the time, to think about the nuances of the language I use. I have to realise that black voices can conflict, there is no 'black narrative' only all the black voices, which may themselves seem to conflict and disagree and yet still be valid. It doesn't have to be simple for us, easy to understand. We just need to listen, even when it's uncomfortable. Especially then. And this is good advice in the face of any discrimination. I'm not sure loads of people, men especially made this journey though. If you're sitting next to one, maybe have a chat about it. [4]

---

[4] If you're a man, especially a white man, reading this book, you might feel a couple of things. First off blamed for something you didn't do. Most men I know are nice, kind, compassionate ones without a conscious agenda to play into these problems. Secondly like I must be one of those raving feminists - a man-hater. It's not that. It's just that we *need* your help. There are problems in the world that you maybe aren't privy to or you don't step in to defend because they don't necessarily effect you, you've not been paying attention. And that needs to change, please. Do the work stop laughing at the jokes. Doing nothing, isn't helping.

Body Stories
Kerrie Rycroft

She/Her, Anti-racist, Single Mum, Opinionated and Proud of it

Reproduced with permission.

Facebook 9th June 2020

Hey white local friends, I have some questions for you. Don't worry, Facebook's special algorithms won't show many of you this post, it knows you're hugely uncomfortable and will only show you the cute pony posts and the ones asking what I should watch on Netflix. You can carry on your life comfortably pretending racism only happens in America.

As you were...

Have you ever walked into a pub with your kids and had two grown men in their 40s turn up their noses, laugh and say 'suddenly smells bad in here' as your children walk past their table? I have - Paul Pry in Peterborough, June 2019

What about sat in Pizza Hut in Grantham, Peterborough, Huntingdon or in Nandos in Lincoln and Huntingdon or The Harvester in Boston and had a nice white family of four refuse to sit next to you or ask to be moved somewhere different?

Have you ever sat in the Wellhead Park in Bourne watching your children play and had a dad walk up with his two children and tell them not to go near your kids while they play, or else?

What about that lovely lady in Folkingham who makes stained glass, ever been there to buy a present to hear a story about her family who moved up from London 'to get away from the blacks' but she is not racist, she didn't mean the blacks like *my* children, she meant those other ones. The horrible ones. She is sure my children are lovely. So that's OK, right?

Ever been into Co-op at Morton and been asked where you adopted your children from and then had the person express shock that you gave birth to them because they look so different from you, how strange.

How many times has your son been racially abused in one year at school - and we're talking times that were so bad they actually got reported rather than just the shit that goes on in the playground? Nine. In one year. Two of them bad enough that the bus driver reported them.

Has your daughter ever started at a new secondary school to find that all her classmates say her name in a strong African accent whenever the teachers aren't around? Trinity has such a ring to it when said in a way that's meant as a social slur don't you think? Took her weeks to be brave enough to tell me and almost as long to get them to stop.

Talking of schools has your child ever been asked to choose if they are black or white, because both is not an option on the school admissions form? Come on now don't be greedy, which one ARE you? What part of your rich heritage will you drop when you put this blazer on?

Or has your child ever had written 'due to his ethic background and family situation, Cameron is deemed to be a high-risk student and caution should be taken on the walk home with his friends' about them on their first week at school?

Do people stare at you when you are out with your children?

Are people unable to hide their surprise when they meet your children for the first time?

How many times have you heard someone say - ooohh all from the same dad, that's rare for someone like him.

How many of your children would have stuck up for mine in any of the above circumstances?
How many of your children even know what's going on in the world?
Have you ever sat down with your children and explained to them that the gorgeous colour of their skin comes with a price tag. That they need to be careful. That they will be judged and found to be both too black and too white by the same white people.

How can I expect the whole world to change when my tiny corner of it won't?
If you made it this far - you can share xx

Then the 2020 'Obesity Crisis'

It felt like every month brought a new sideswipe. *Fat people are dying from the Coronavirus! What about the Obesity Crisis!* There isn't one. Politicians and the media have invented a fakestorm. I'll explain more…

In his book, *The Truth About Fat* Anthony Warner explains:

The impact of weight gain, 'in terms of health outcomes for most people is largely irrelevant'.

'There will never be a one-size-fits-all solution, yet that is what we crave, and that is what is constantly being searched for. As a result, people genuinely in need of help are cast aside as wide-reaching interventions are designed on the premise that they might shave tiny amounts of weight from the whole population. In trying to 'cure' everyone of these few extra pounds, we are actually helping no one… In reality, those people that extreme obesity affects form a small minority' (2.5% of the population over 40 BMI).

'The term (obesity) 'epidemic' is unhelpful at best, frequently leveraged for political gain, with the potential to hurt a great many people. It has added to the demonisation of fat people on a worldwide scale.'[145]

If truly we are concerned about an 'obesity crisis', then as in the chapter *How We're Making People Fat*, how we behave and conduct ourselves around that perceived problem is the exact opposite of what would help the situation.

Let me share with you my letter to Secretary of State for Health and Social Care, Matt Hancock during the 'obesity crisis' of 2020.

Dear Mr Hancock

I am writing in regard to the recent news reports that obesity is linked to death rates due to Covid 19. I am aware that there is a plan being devised this week in response.

I run a business called BodEquality and it is a world-first in that it educates organisations around body image and the many factors influencing why our bodies present the way they do and what might constitute meaningful change in terms of progress.

One thing that largely doesn't help a fat person is a sense of social rejection, shame, judgement.

Negative body image impacts 91% of women and 40+% of men. Can lead to depression, self-harm, low self-regard and suicide. 13% of adults are reported to have considered suicide based on their body image - (how they feel about their body). Anorexia is the largest killer of all the psychiatric illnesses. And yet we still use the same out-dated approaches to address the 'obesity issue'.

Eat less, move more, shame fat. There is very little narrative about mental weight (the effort we waste worrying about weight that rarely changes); or mental ill health and its impact on weight, childhood trauma / disability / injury and weight outcomes.

The current approach to weight is so simplistic as to be pretty useless. We need to change the conversation and go deep into the factors influencing people's relationships with their bodies. As a society much like as individuals, in order to forge change, we need to harness some compassion.

My course would offer a quick way of MPs appraising the evidence here. Of educating people to shift their mindsets to a more enlightened approach, sure to reap a more successful response.

If I could change one thing, it would be the sensationalist and shaming nature that fat people are depicted and targeted in our press and clearly still in our policy-making.

If I can be of any help, please do let me know.

All the best

Emi Howe BSc. Cert. Ed. M.F.H.T.

I also emailed 21 further MPs, All Party Parliamentary Groups for: Body Image, Obesity, Eating Disorders, multiple media outlets and the press office for the Department of Health and Social Care. You know what happened? You already know it. Nothing. The ravings of a mad woman…

How To Help A Fat Person

A Blog published July 2020 – BodEquality.com

It's really simple, don't. At least not in the traditional way. Not in the way we've become accustomed to and has been highlighted by yet another 'obesity crisis' in the media - this time with a Covid twist.

What the government is marketing as a 'world-leading plan', claiming 'These bold measures will help us tip the scales on obesity. The argument for action is the clearest it's ever been.'

Aside from how inappropriate the term 'tip the scales' is, hon, it doesn't matter how clear the argument for action is, if the action doesn't or can't yield results. There I've said it. It's the biggest load of hokum I've seen since I last saw BoJo downing a kale smoothie.

Don't help fat people by making them feel: like a failure, ashamed, judged, wrong, incapable, stupid, invisible, patronised, unhealthy, scared, in danger, powerless, excluded.

I've grown up with a Mum who has been 'morbidly obese' for my whole life – I learnt that term as a young child. I'm now 41 and am wondering if it was a misnomer because she's far outlived my slim gym-going father. What I have witnessed over the years is her simple inability to lose weight. She just can't. Now in her 70's with limited mobility, I'm certain she won't in the time and to the level expected by Matt Hancock MP - the press release from gov.uk urges us to 'lose weight to beat coronavirus'. Mum's relationship with her body is multi-dimensional, as it is for all of us. Telling her she's at higher risk now, just serves to scare her, positioning her weight loss as instrumental to us beating coronavirus, will likely send her straight to the fridge.

You know, research shows some people just drew the long straw when bodies were being handed out. We may find it easier to be thin, that doesn't make us experts. Doing varied research makes experts.

What I know from Mum and from those I've interviewed for my work, is that such shame can be felt around fat bodies as to make it a subject that is agony to broach, even to themselves. No, thankfully, it hasn't killed her, just made her life less. A lot less.

During the current obesity sham, as a response, the Department for Health and Social Care have taken to twitter and offered a stirring 24 second film entitled 'Obesity Makes Us Vulnerable'.

Let's see what's going on over on the NHS website dedicated to 'better health'. As expected, under the title 'Kickstart Your Health' we have nods to BMI, calories, meal planning and weight-loss goals. Eat less, move more, lose weight. That is health. No… just that isn't health.

Meanwhile anyone (such as the charity Mind) calling for the need to reduce the stigma around mental health are going to be left wanting. Mental health has been given exactly zero airtime on this subject and let's remember, the subject is health. I scroll down the NHS 'better health' website to find a quiz entitled 'How are you?'. A glimmer of hope, but alas, it asked me if I'd rather eat ham than a burger, to ignore my (temporary) disability and focus on what I eat instead (dear God), it then gave me a health score of 6/10 and some handy tips around moving, eating, drinking and smoking. So not really 'how are you', more… *what* are you.

And it's a hoax - another one. What it actually amounts to is 'statistics show nearly 8% of critically ill patients in intensive care units with coronavirus have been morbidly obese, compared with 2.9% of the general population'[146] - who are 'morbidly obese'. These stats have been used in such a skewed way as to be transformed into 'fat people will die of Covid' - not even all 'morbidly obese' people will die of Covid. They have a higher chance, but they still account for less than 8% of critically ill Covid patients. Care Minister Helen Whately, who appears to benefit from thin privilege, speaking on BBC News:

'Most people don't want to be overweight, it's just hard to make those choices that would make you lose weight and one of the things is, becoming overweight doesn't happen overnight, it's a consequence of over an extended period of time, eating a little bit extra, for many, many days at a time so it's something that builds up gradually over time. And losing weight is about changing those habits and we want to give people the information, the support so that they can do what many people want to do.'

...injury, metabolism, leptin levels - in fact 25 genes now linked to obesity, socioeconomics, childhood trauma, exercise anxiety, eating disorders, lack of privilege...

We aren't in the midst of an 'obesity time bomb'. Again, the population's weight has increased steadily and proportionately in accordance with height and income since the 1920s. In that time, the natural variance and diversity in bodies hasn't changed, despite all our efforts.

Something else that has happened since the 1920s, as the government's own website through the Office of National Statistics shows, is a clear increase in life expectancy. So all the scaremongering about worsening outcomes in the face of cancer, diabetes and now Covid-19, really only amount to one thing. The one thing we are so fearful of, we'll try anything to avoid it. That one thing is the cold hard truth that... we all will die. We can't avoid it, no matter what body we're in. As a cancer survivor, I don't take that truth lightly. But by their own admission, we are living longer and longer.

In reality the group of people this impacts is the extreme of obesity - 2.9% of society make up the group that might need some very specific multi-dimensional approaches to initiate positive change. For example this might be counselling around a binge eating disorder or tackling childhood trauma. Maybe we could spend the 'better health' budget on that?

From many academic researchers before me, we know that our mental health has a massive impact on our eating and exercising behaviours. As The Mental Health Foundation pointed out during Mental Health Awareness Week in 2019, having negative feelings about our bodies is linked to: depression, self harm, suicide and unhealthy eating practices. So adding more fuel to that fire, by condemning fat people under this Covid umbrella is misplaced.

We know that crash dieting is more likely to result in weight yoyoing and ultimately a higher BMI than we started with, or at the other extreme, an eating disorder. You could argue that by making a show of fat people in this way, the message compounds the problem.

I don't mean to nit-pick, it's just this trajectory is now dated. Which would be fine if it worked but it hasn't worked in the past; it won't work now. We've got an opportunity to get smarter and put some genuine thought into it. Or at least stop doing this while the research strongly advocates against it. It's not just that its dated, it's that it's uninformed, unevolved and comes at a cost to individuals and organisations.

Progress looks like treating people as individuals. Empowering people and their: choices, history, genetics, abilities, allowing them their story. We can offer ourselves acceptance, compassion and encouragement and extend it to those around us. That may induce weight loss, it may not.

What if we try the opposite of obesity scaremongering, compassion on a social scale. Letting people know, they can be who they are, that they are valuable, empowered to be who and how they want, their health is their business. Avoid focussing on early death rates; none of us can control when we're going to die - but this rhetoric is stealing our life. It is creating barriers to change for certain people, not well-meaning life rafts.

And as for the 8% - BoJo needs to pump some money into the NHS to deal with it. To take responsibility and stop blaming a natural and historical social trend.

Postscript Mum says: 'What I don't understand is that people think I *want* to be like this! You've got this spot on, thank you for understanding.'

Post Postscript: One of my lovely first readers reflected with the following note: 'While I totally agree with all the observations and comments in this section, I feel it is important still to acknowledge the impact obesity has on the lives of those who live with it and around it and the hidden cost to the NHS through diabetes, heart conditions, mobility problems etc. These are genuine concerns that should be addressed but with no shame attached. Hope that's not too controversial!'

This is one of the concerns that has and is going to come up in many people so, with permission, I explore it here.

Reader: I nearly didn't mention anything but it kept coming back to me that if we're not careful the whole message of not judging and shaming any body shape and size, while essentially being the absolutely right thing to do, can cross the line into saying that they're OK with having no responsibility to at least be healthy and not expect the NHS to 'fix' their lifestyle choices when it leads to ill health. Such a tricky one, and I really don't mean it to be offensive or prejudiced in any way, just that I do believe that we all have a responsibility to try to maintain all aspects of our health, and expect the NHS to be there to help us when needed but not to simply 'do it all for us' with no responsibility on our part to do the work needed. It's such a fascinating subject.

Emi: I'm writing my email, I'm worried it might come off a bit harsh. I'm trying to soften it.

Reader: Oh please don't worry, that's why I hesitated about my note as I don't want to sound like I'm blaming people for their obesity! Send what you feel and we can work from there.

My email: To what end is it important to acknowledge the personal and NHS cost of obesity? I believe part of this dialogue is still wrapped up in The Glitch, where obesity is perceived as a problem that we can eradicate. We don't need to acknowledge the personal impact - those living with obesity know the impact it has on them and wider awareness of it isn't low.
The NHS obesity cost isn't actually that hidden, you may be mentioning it here, precisely because it isn't hidden. We hear about it through the news and media all the time, perhaps we're conditioned to be concerned about it. Actual hidden costs might be the ones associated with eating disorders (£4.6 billion) that we never hear about but equally, what are the hidden costs of broken limbs? The NHS is there to serve the nation's health problems, whatever form they come in. We're all living longer, is that also a drain? As I hope I've outlined, obesity is most often not a conscious choice. So what benefit does acknowledging its cost above say a fracture clinic's cost. The National Health Service is one designed to support the health of our natural, diverse society, not a fictional society

where everyone is thin or health is only aligned with thinness. Alienating certain demographics as draining it, can't be separated from a narrative of blame. In the chapter *How We're Making People Fat* there's a strong argument for shifting our social focus from blame to empowerment. Who knows, maybe then the cost may start to diminish, but as a bi-product of centring and supporting *people* first.

Reader: Goodness this is hard! As soon as I've put something down on paper and look back on it I can see immediately how my choice of words is wrong! 'Lifestyle choices' is such a bad description which suggests I feel obese people are choosing that lifestyle… I'm certainly not. I think I'm trying to say that maybe we do have a choice in whether to seek help and do our part in the necessary journey to 'improve our health' as a general part of society. Now that is assuming of course that such help is available and accessible, which we all know in the case of mental health it definitely isn't at least not on the scale it needs to be, which is a huge part of the problem here.

You are absolutely right about the other costs to the NHS, fractures for example. If we suffered repeated injuries from the type of sport we played, should we be refused treatment? No but I do still feel that we all have to accept some responsibility for what we expect the NHS to fix, and we can't just carry on doing the wrong things to our bodies. Even now I'm not sure I've put this across in the right way Emi.

Emi: I would say, any pressure to 'perform health' for society is not an effective or positive motivator for health and for some might even antagonise the issue.

Reader: But personal responsibility is, I feel still important simply to be as 'healthy' as we can be. This is such an emotive subject Emi and I certainly don't want to come across as not understanding or agreeing with the bigger picture here, because I absolutely do.

Emi: I know this kind of dialogue is tough, thank you for sticking with it. I think perhaps there's just more unlearning to do, that's all. Without walking in another's shoes we run the risk of viewing it through our prism of privilege. We can't know how accessible taking that physical responsibility is, even if people desperately want to. Or how social pressure to take the responsibility adds mentally and emotionally to the problem when more pressing things are involved. It again prides and values physical health as the pinnacle of health while mental and emotional health are ignored. We have so long been sold the fat lazy dialogue. If the barrier is lack of money, self-assurance, a childhood abuse trauma and fear of being seen as attractive or an internal feeling so empty that only food abates it or brings any relief, it positions it differently. These are the questions which naturally rise through the process of looking at bodies differently and maybe an aspect that we won't fully agree on. It's OK it we don't. It's meant only to show another way of looking at it. I think you've raised a valid point that needs addressing, that it may discourage some people from going after their best achievable health. I think that's what you mean and maybe that needs highlighting more? What you're offering here is so valuable because you won't be alone in doubting this and these sorts of questions do start forming for many as we start to think differently.

Reader: When I read all you've said I totally agree with and do understand and empathise - I do not want to come across as preachy or taking a moral high ground - but then I am as you point out in the book thin-privileged. I wish with all my heart that the right help was there for everyone but maybe I'm missing the point in that you might add 'should they want it?' And if they don't is that ok, when the result may arguably end in high costs to an already overstretched service? But maybe that's the problem - I maybe unthinkingly added that comment at the end of the section dealing with fat shaming and so it feels I'm targeting obesity as the problem here. I really didn't mean that, my issue is general responsibility across the board. Years ago, when my two were babies, a friend was told that if she asked for it her G.P. would give her Calpol on prescription. Her husband was a bank manager, both well off, but she took it. My own parents insisted on asking for prescriptions for paracetamol, etc, when it costs peanuts in the supermarket (they probably thought the ones the G.P. gave them were 'better' than the ones I bought them!) Personal responsibility to not take NHS resources when they are not necessary would leave more resources for mental health and I think that's where my point was maybe not well explained. If everyone took a little more personal responsibility then there might be more money for mental health resources. I really don't want to come across as not understanding the mental anguish and long-standing trauma behind all of these issues. A different take can be seen as helpful but not if I have worded it in such as way that I seem dismissive or condescending, then I haven't explained myself well at all. You're so right when you say it needs so much more discussion, which hopefully will result from your amazing work. Don't know if I've made this any clearer or just muddied the waters! But I like to think it's not about agreeing or disagreeing, just both (and all) of us trying to learn more.

Emi: It's not just a case of 'if they want it', it's also if it's accessible or even *possible*. It might not be through: disability, injury, limiting lifelong beliefs, an eating disorder… Remember our 'best health' isn't a basic need like food and shelter. Many other needs come before being able to assimilate our 'best health'.

Everything you're saying is all valid and only what I know many other people will also be thinking and thanking you for bringing up. Having spent years absorbing body positive messages, you could argue, I am conditioned to that view too.

However, I hope I don't sound condescending, and I might be wrong, there are ideas in this book (and this is why this dialogue is so important) that are probably really new for you. What I am hearing is you tussling with two strongly held belief systems. The new and the old. It is totally natural, your questions are ones I had to ask along the way too. I believe everyone does. But here's the thing, in the case of obesity, the traditional medical model *isn't* working. It isn't 'curing', reducing or even stabilising it. Like thin pressure imagery, social health pressure is abstract and doesn't serve as a personal health motivator. Deep personal reasons to go after our own health, tied to our own self-worth are, in my experience, what motivates health.

I'm concerned that perhaps a really important part of what I'm trying to get across is being missed. That is to give people their bodies and body choices back to them, no strings attached. No directive to follow. Allow them to connect with their own bodies and from there build a level of health they feel comfortable with. That may focus more on mental health and reducing stress and won't look like what we've been trained to see as health, but it is still better health to them.

I do appreciate all concerns around adding more pressure to the NHS by perceiving this as effectively allowing people to opt out of health if they want to. It might. But it also might empower people to go after a realistic health that is within grasp.

I think if any of this is ringing true, it might be worth giving this book another read. I've certainly done that in the past with books that I've felt have changed me and are deserving of more of my attention to really get to grips with new ideas. If these concepts are new, you won't be the same persona at the end of reading it as you were at the beginning and so reading it again, you may have a different experience.

What you are doing is giving this deep thought and allowing it to shift your internal landscape. It's not always easy. And I might be wrong and in three years time you might still feel the same way. What I think we can agree on is more needs to be spent to raise the profile of mental and emotional health in the NHS and as a service it certainly deserves more funding (please give the nurses a proper pay rise Boris!)

The following day we met up and talked it over. We hashed over some of the same things and Reader was sure she wouldn't feel any differently in the future, she feels really strongly about the role we play in our social responsibility of this issue. We did get down to some really interesting semantics though. Reader kept coming back to the sentence 'It is our social responsibility to help them.' I think at one point I said flatly, 'No it isn't!' I also said 'We can't take personal or social responsibility for fat people without also blaming / judging them.'

Distilling it further Reader conceded maybe *we* don't but doctors do. Perhaps – and done in the right way, without triggering harmful memories or using tactless talk. But not *us*, not society. However further probing revealed that it reflected in Reader more a desire to help people having problems, not just these problems, and that's a very natural instinct and one that feels right on many levels. I kept offering situations where it's not that simple, eating disorders or injury. I was thinking in my head, maybe Reader means a certain type of fat person.

Reader: 'There are people who actively want to be fat.'

Emi: 'I'd say very few'

Reader: 'And there are people who might not know where to go for help.'

Emi: 'But *they* do need to go for help. It's *their* choice and power. Also that help isn't going to disappear because of this book. There will still be people both appropriately and inappropriately helping fat people.'

Reader: Take for example my shoulder op, my doctor was clear to me, he could do the mechanical work of fixing it, but it was up to me to do the exercises to gain back the range of movement. It was my responsibility to regain my health.

Emi: I agree. I felt a responsibility to get healthy too after my diagnosis. But not for the NHS or society, for myself and my family.

Reader: But you see some people don't… My Mum wouldn't. She wanted everything done for her.

Emi: But *you* wanting her to, wouldn't change her.

Reader: (pause) No… you're right! It didn't.

Emi: One of the drives that made me write this book was my Mum. I've lived with her trying to lose weight for 42 years, unsuccessfully. I wish I could take all of that trying, that energy, that attention, the disappointments, the perceived failure, the low self-worth and catapult it into the horizon. I wish instead of her mother teaching her she wasn't good enough that way, she had taught her, no matter what, that she was good enough.

Reader: I used to get so frustrated with my parents, they just weren't active, couldn't even walk the short, flat route to pick up a paper. They just didn't try.

Emi: So when you talk about 'them'.

Reader: Yes… I really mean… my parents.

I sent this over to Reader to check they were happy with it.

Reader: Yes I think this lays out our dialogue well, although doesn't really expand on all the conversation and discussions we had this morning, probably because there just aren't enough pages for that! I've been going over it again and think that what I was trying to put across is that we should still be able to discuss weight issues, if that is a contributory factor to wider health problems, both physical AND mental, without fear of being accused of fat shaming, judging or blaming. We would discuss other lifestyle factors, smoking, drinking, exercise levels, etc., but if we are not allowed to discuss weight then are we truly able to help that person in the best possible way? (here I can hear you saying 'who is "we" and "what if they don't want our help"'! But let's just go with at some point they MIGHT need that help, either physically or mentally, and whoever is trying to help them should feel able to discuss that subject (weight) if it is contributing to their situation.
Goodness that took some thinking through!

Emi: I think this makes for a great conclusion, it shows beautifully how it brings up all these complicated feelings that can be hard to articulate but possible to if we don't give up! Thank you!

Reader: Bless you, I felt it summed up how, though we both may have been coming at it from a different viewpoint, through discussion and listening to each other's experiences and opinions, we arrive at some, even if it isn't all, common ground.

Post, Post Postscript: This is gooey! Since I've finished this book, the two people who have read it so far, have also had slight emotional fall outs from it. I think they can also be described as lightbulb moments. It can be a lot. It can bring up stuff. I'm still not saying I'm right and Reader is wrong. I'm saying, let's talk about it among our friends, let's hash it out. Where are those feelings coming from? Let's seek talking therapy if it feels right. There will be questions and that's natural. And it's OK to disagree, it's OK to change, or stay the same. As for anyone, this has to be driven by you.

Seeing 2020

I had gathered my BodEquality Course Market Research:

- Did you find the course valuable? 100% answered: Yes
- Would you recommend this course to others? 100% answered: Yes
- 'It's a great short course and introduction to the world of body image and coupled with the downloads, is an excellent resource pack. I think employers should definitely offer this as part of their health and wellbeing provisions. A real value-for-money investment for organisations' Runa, Time to Change, MIND
- 'BodEquality is a well presented and thought-provoking course. It covers an important topic around the perception of body image, which Business as a whole, needs to reflect and take notice of.' Nick Butcher, HR Strategy Pro
- 'This course taught me not to talk about my weight so much. Me my family and friends are all guilty of it' Anon
- 'I love it, the stories from the diverse individuals brings home the fact it's not just certain individuals this may affect, it is in fact all kinds of people.' Joe
- 'It's a great initiative, haven't come across anything similar. Any organisation / workplace would definitely benefit from this.' Maria Katsarou, Counsellor
- 'It will make me more respectful of the wide range of behaviours, thoughts and feelings body image can bring up, both consciously and unconsciously.' Steve Loft

It became clear that employers have no idea the human cost a negative body image can have. Again because being negative about our bodies has become absorbed into modern culture as to be virtually invisible. We live simultaneously acknowledging the fakery of the media, while demanding the impossible of our bodies, with very little to rationalise the gap. The BodEquality course is a tool that can fill that gap and address the wider issues in the workplace.

Research tells us that 'body talk' is a common workplace distraction, according to Udemy in 2018, 66% of workers hadn't spoken to their managers about office distractions, 31% would like businesses to define cultural norms around distractions at work.[147] In-house body talk alienates team members – more people than you might imagine. Impacting their mental health, their eating and exercising habits and their output and sick day quota.

As the summer progressed, I started to reach out to companies, to engage people with my work. Later I created an autumn newsletter, stating the case for BodEquality in business. It talked about how having a positive self-regard at work can have positive returns for business. Remember those stats from Anglican Water - an eight-fold benefit after centring wellbeing at work.[148] The newsletter also dealt with avoiding losses or wasting company time, companies' Public Sector Equality Duty, all things that the course addresses.

Finally it looked at The Chartered Institute of Personnel and Development's Wellbeing at Work, Survey Report, March 2020.[149] Their Wellbeing Model acknowledges five domains of wellbeing including: Health, Work, Personal Growth, Social/Collective and Values and Principles. Body image dissatisfaction impacts all of them. It further highlighted their findings of The Impact and Effectiveness of Well-being Initiatives where wellbeing initiatives were linked positively to employee engagement and reduction of sick days.

The newsletter included, with permission, a case study of a LinkedIn post, shared by Jessica Joan Richards, whose post about workplace body shaming went viral at the time, received almost 39,000 comments and was viewed 19 million times. I'd demonstrated, the very current and relevant nature of this subject.

I created a *How Do You Feel About Your Body* – flow chart to help it resonate with HR folks. I made a quiz, urging them to think about it when perhaps in the past they never have in the context of work…

Age 41

Last year I made a promise to my husband that my BodEquality work would pay off in twelve months or I would stop doing it (giving my time and our money to it) and go and get a proper job. My promise ran out in June. It's now October 2020. We are mid Covid. My promise did *not* see this coming. Twelve months ago I'd never even heard of Covid. My computer is giving the word a squiggley red underline because it doesn't know it either!

Some people meet lack of control with food control and stop eating. Some people meet it the other way and try and fill the hole. And some people do neither. That is the natural way of real and diverse bodies. That is also where I am right now. Fatter. But I still love my body. What's more, I don't have the resources actually to do anything else. To monitor every food and movement transaction, I've got more important things to do, more interesting things actually.

Covid weight gain

Panic: Let me in!

Self-preservation: Do NOT let them in.

Excitement: Oh God, what's going on?

Doubt: The Anxiety Squad are trying to get in. Should we let them in?

Vanity: Ambition! You'll listen. This has gone *too* far.

Doubt: They might be right though.

Self-preservation: They're not! How many times have we done this dance before.

Fear: But, we're getting FAT!

Self-preservation: I know. You're right and I do hear you. It's not like we're here in behaviour HQ not noticing. It's just…

Panic: Just what?

Ambition: It's just… and I know you mean well, but you guys, you don't help. You mean to, I know, but you just actually…

Excitement: Make it worse?

Ambition: Yes.

Vanity: You do realise we can't fit into the lazy day jeans any more. You know the big ones!

Panic: She's put them in the loft!

Fear: *And* she threw away the scales so we don't even know how…!

Doubt: I mean *that* is a point.

Self-preservation: We've got it *handled.* Give us time. If we try and fix this right now, we'll end up crashing again and you remember the crash of 2003 don't you?

Fear: But what about her health?

Optimism: Don't worry, we are still strong with the healthy messaging. There are more pressing threats to her health right now.

Self-preservation: Like staying sane while trying to work from home, deal with an invisible virus and home-school the kids, it's just… more immediate.

Panic: How can you be so calm?
Self-preservation: Because we've been here before, we know what to do. She needs to be in the right frame of mind, and life needs to be more… manageable, that's all. Just give us all some time.
Optimism: Guys, I've got to agree on this. Every time you lot stick your oar in, it just gets uncomfortable, and that's what we're trying to avoid right now. It doesn't help, even though you *really* think it does.
Ambition: *Please*, can you go back to your stations. Those eyebrows won't pluck themselves, and heaven knows what scrapes we've got into while the motor-reflex has been unmanned!

A Long View Reflection of The Petition

I think it's fair to say that the petition didn't work and I've put a lot of thought into why. My conclusions fall into three categories.

1. Apathy, we're too busy with our lives (and comfortable) to be bothered to take action – and so many petitions are making the rounds these days.
2. Most people don't see the problem or the need for anything to change – don't recognise is as a 'real' problem.
3. Most people don't believe it can or will ever change.

But there were other forces at play. I also learned that many people, especially in my generation, really struggle with the idea of loving their bodies and I was conscious of creating yet another impossible standard. Such heavy programming might stand between us and a tick on a petition. I have a chequered history of ups and downs in the route to loving my body. I remember what it felt like. That it can feel impossible. This is something that Godmother of Body Image, Kim Chernin also reflected on towards the end of her career.

Chernin's work was about body and appetite acceptance, in the landscape of a patriarchy fearing bigger female bodies and trying to shrink our power. If a patient came to her wanting to lose weight, she would often refer them on to another clinician. However, writing in 2013, Chernin looked back over her career with some regret, she acknowledged that perhaps she had been 'close-minded' and 'my earlier ideas were hardening into an absolute, as if what was right for some women had to be right for *all* women, another one-size-fits-all approach to women and food.' [150]

While I'm fully in support of accepting our bodies exactly as they are and not feeling any pressure to lose weight, for mental health and self-agency purposes, and am an advocate of valuing real bodies, the natural diversity of bodies etc. can we also not alienate people who might *want* to diet, who feel safe with a plan or a system relating to food. Lizzo recently received backlash from the BoPo community after sharing her ten-day smoothie diet. She responded: 'I feel like as a big girl, people just expect if you are doing something for health you're doing it for dramatic weight loss, and that is not the case.' Reiterating that 'every big girl should do whatever they want with their bodies.' [151]

I got myself in a fairly complicated lexicon with The Girl One recently who was baffled by me bad-mouthing 'diets' but then I launched straight into: 'It's just not that healthy to cut things completely from our diets.' She was outraged, 'You just said it's bad to diet!'

Yes we use 'diet' in terms of simply, our relationship with food. You might argue, there is no getting away from it. Even in the sphere of 'non-diets' or intuitive eating, we still have to eat, it's very hard to erase the programming we've received about food beliefs and rules, even if we're trying to break those rules, it's still a system.

Chernin talked about using diets as a therapeutic tool and in some instances using the emotions they bring up to access and process long-term underlying mental health issues[152]. Also that our 'hunger' might not be for food but for other passions we've been repressed from pursuing – it's thought-provoking stuff.

I was also annoyed at how creating petition content, was making me overthink things, edit and stage things, in order to have 'the optics' to be noticeable – the opposite of what I stand for – it is a job, a craft and there are those who do it so well while also acknowledging the glitch but it takes time and thought.

I start to wonder what it takes to truly create a drastic shift such as this. What I needed was a stunt. Should I have gathered some people to sit naked outside the ASA with me and call the papers? My friends are loyal and true but that might be asking a bit much, even for them! I think back to the suffragettes and ask myself, is someone going to have to publicly die, to create this shift? After all they already are, just very privately.

Awkward Conversations

How We Killed Diana (You, Me and Us)

I just have this sinking feeling that we're wandering through the modern world, not really paying any attention to the fact that we've created a culture that is really messing us up! So much of our media and advertising is at best contrived, suggestive, at worst misleading and damaging to health and almost always fantasy. In the name of a 'free press', we have a largely unregulated media. But as I've hopefully demonstrated, we don't have a free press. The press are on an agenda, interested in churning out contrived, self-serving propaganda, often tapping into people's worst instincts and affirming them. Perhaps there is no place in the traditional media for my voice or similar voices - as I know others have struggled too. I also know others still who have had to compromise their authenticity to play to the press, and not tackle this issue. It is an echo chamber of the dominant unequal (white/male/commercial) narrative. Creating problems where there were none, to sell stories. For every click on a scare-mongering headline, snarky article, gossipy commentary, celebrity non-story, we read, for every paparazzi that hounds down a princess, we contribute to it simply because we don't stop looking at it, clicking on it buying it.

How can you inform people about a story that they might care about and let them know *why* they should care, if you can't find your way into the vehicle that shares stories? While also, that vehicle is accountable for the problem you'd like to talk about?

I suspect Credos - the UK advertising's think tank - was right when they assured me the only way things will change, is through consumer pressure. I suspect that if we want The Glitch to change, if we want the media to change, if we want the law to change or The Equality Act to change, or the CAP codes to change, if we want visibility in branding to change, or the NHS to change, or the Directors or the attitudes of the ASA to change, if you want the Financial Controllers of fashion retailers to change, (did you realise how many cogs were turning in this Glitch?) If you want your kids to change… I truly believe, the only way all of that will change is if we change. You, me and us.

When you're lying in a hospital bed, wondering if your second baby will make it, or your third, or fourth. When you're lying in a hospital bed, wondering if *you* will make it, you realise – this is it. There's not more than this. It's fake, a lie. The best use of your time would actually be to find a way to love this life, this body, this reality and stop searching for something else. You can either enjoy and find joy and worth in this and the people you share this with, or not. Because there is nothing else. This is it. In this final week of pulling the book together I received the news, such sad news, that Cathy, my long-time client had gone. Cathy was so much more than just a client - she had been at my wedding, helped make the flowers, had been at my Boobie Shower. She was my friend and her energy, positivity and bravery will be so missed. Within hours I learned that another lovely client, Claire had also lost her cancer battle.

It's only about love, people and contribution.

Nothing else really matters, when the time comes. Certainly no one will care about your body… other than it's gone. I've made myself cry now…

What Change Doesn't Mean

- Don't stop going after your health, supporting your body, nurturing it, giving it what it needs within the parameters our personal lives gives us. Connect with your body feelings regularly and listen to what it wants, how you can help it.

- Don't stop making up, feeling beautiful, painting nails, doing hair, whatever it is that makes you feel great. Do all of it, to any level but do it for you, for your self-care reasons, do it because there's wellbeing in it, there's connection and energy and spirit attached to looking and feeling your best. But don't do it because the marketing made you feel anything other than 'enough, exactly as you are'.

- It doesn't mean not noticing people's bodies. Noticing is not the same as judging.

- It doesn't mean never thinking or saying another negative body thing again (don't panic). This is a process, a muscle that will get stronger.

Change Looks Like

- Authenticity and acceptance. It means developing a deep connection and appreciation of our magical, awe-inspiring bodies that isn't simply 'Oh my God, delete that photo!'

- Changing where we put our attention and what we believe about bodies.

- Changing where we spend our money.

- We need to show them *We Value Reality*. Demanding more reality and integrity from our media and ads and talk with our wallets, our attention and our time.

- Whenever you get the urge to change, that you're not enough as you are, ask if anyone would profit from that feeling. Have you been sold it?

- Check our click-reflex. Just take a beat before you click on social / traditional media and give it precious moments of your life. This system is not set up for our benefit. For every reinforcement of false ideals, it hurts us bit by bit by imperceptible, damaging bit. Follow @BodEquality for regular reality checks and inspiration of accounts to follow to increase your reality quota.

- We know all of this! We just haven't paid it enough attention to internalise it – we haven't cleared a path in our neural pathways - because clearly it still works! We need to demand more.

- We can ask ourselves, now that we've freed up this extra time, money, energy, confidence, what do we really want? What are the questions we want answering? What positive impact can we have? What interests can we pursue, what talents can we develop? What are we going to do with our extra power?

- We can change in our homes, our workplaces, or social groups. We can rise and bring others with us, what can we do to raise the consciousness around The Glitch? To evolve not just our self-image but also our communities?

- We need to hear this message relentlessly if we're to redress the balance and if the world isn't going to provide it then we must. We must be relentlessly real.

In Conclusion

One of the reasons I wrote this book is because whenever one of my friends bad-mouthed their bodies, I had a tendency to overwhelm them (quite passionately I might add) with my need for them to have all of this information in their head (sorry friends). Now I can stop that, and just give them this book. Phew!

On one level I do feel satisfied. Nothing much has changed in fact, but me. What has changed in me is that I no longer have questions about why I felt that way about my body. Or why we live in this weird duality scam. Fifteen-year-old me has had questions that she couldn't even vocalise, answered. And on some level that feels like progress. I honestly thought there was nothing I could do, and yet… I've done this!

In case I haven't been too clear, living next to, enmeshed with, yet still disconnected from this crazy fantasy world poses a real harm to our health, to our lives. Progress has to start with us. You, me and us. All of us. I can see clearly now, how the world isn't ethical, kind, inclusive; it is only commercial. Seeing it in these terms makes me so sad. Makes me ready to move on to the next era. I have no doubt that the future will ridicule us for The Glitch. I also predict the future will incorporate our energy, feelings and the mind-body connection and its health potential into just about everything. We have ignored and pooh-poohed it to our detriment.

We are the customer of the globe. We define what the standard needs to be. And instead of thanklessly reaching for an impossible standard, how about we create a real standard, still high, based on kindness, empathy, compassion, understanding, suspended judgement, and inclusion. Recognising and validating everyone's experience. Us rising collectively with knowledge and awareness of the reality of bodies, of valuing real bodies, in acknowledging the natural diversity of bodies.

Do I intend this book to be a statement? A call to arms? Well yes. Have I got time to wait for the publishing industry to make it's slow march to possible publication. Nope. I've done it myself. There is no marketing budget. So together, how do we go about creating the widespread shift required? I'm guessing you lot will have some good ideas. Who do you/we need, to have this information in their head?

We can keep learning, read more:

- For a truly magical account of our frankly ridiculously incredible bodies, head over to Bill Bryson's The Body: A Guide for Occupants

- For more stuff about the reality of our diverse bodies I recommend Anthony Warner's The Truth About Fat: Why Obesity is not that Simple.

- To continue your fat education pick up Stephanie Yeboah's Fattily Ever After and Aubrey Gordon's What We Don't Talk About When We Talk About Fat.

- And you'll find many more resources and forward links on the website free resources section. www.bodequality.com

The Valuing Real Bodies Manifesto

- The Equalities Act acknowledging body image, valuing real bodies and honoring the natural diversity of bodies

- This filtered through to all elements of government and via the Advertising Association to the ASA and CAP

- The ASA and CAP being held accountable for modelling inclusion – like every other industry is. What allows certain industries to forego inclusion? Shouldn't inclusion be for everyone, everywhere, if it is to be of any value at all?

- ASA / CAP *reflecting* natural concepts of beauty – they don't get to define it. Beauty comes in all forms and is different for everyone.

- While we're there, a more diverse group of directors for the ASA please. Make the boardroom table bigger.

- For everyone to stop passing the blame.

- I would like body image to be a requirement of the school curriculum in every year group. Taught termly.

- Fatphobia to be viewed as legitimate and abhorrent as homophobia and racism. Again I turn to Anthony Warner

> who highlights the 'vicious stigma that fat people face every day. (We need) to educate the public that this is no longer acceptable. To shout loudly that this abuse is as damaging, illogical and as stupid as any other form of prejudice.'[153]

All of this relies on a culture shift of epic proportions! Widespread awareness and the desire to change at the heart of it. But we're on our way…

Besides over 150 references that help to back up this work, my recommendations aren't stand alone, many of them featured in: The 2016 Body Confidence Event, The Youth Select Committee Report of 2017, were re-iterated in the 2018 ASA public consultation by: The Girl Guides, The Equalities and Human Rights Commission, The National Education Union. Last year in 2020, the Women and Equalities Committee lead an enquiry into poor body image:

'Because it's such a widespread problem, influenced by multiple factors, it's easy to underestimate the real misery it causes – and to so many people. There has been plenty of commentary on the problem, but identifying proposals to tackle it is more challenging. Our inquiry aims to do exactly that: we will be hearing from a wide range of witnesses – both experts and individuals speaking from their own experience, and we will be making recommendations to Government early next year.'[154]

This I understand will address many of my concerns including: The 2010 Equalities Act, the impact of advertising and social media and whether we're 'sufficiently protected from ads that are damaging to body image?' It will outline what steps government could take to improve body image? But will anything change? I hope so. Only time will tell.

Andra Day's Rise Up has been my fight song to help me finish this book, if you're near a streaming device, maybe play it while you read this next bit.

I remember towards the end of the campaign, I came across an image online, a meme. It was of a person at the bottom of a big hole. At the top of the hole was another person, leaning down, stretching out their arms that would clearly never reach with the words 'I wish I could help!' Lying behind them on the ground was a ladder. That's how I truly felt at the end of the campaign. I was at the bottom of that hole, only there wasn't just one person at the top, there were hundreds, thousands maybe millions who could have helped. Having compiled all of my work together (and this is not even all of it) I am staggered by how hard I've worked to try and make a difference. It has cost me in every way. I feel accomplished, proud and done.

What's next? First and foremost let's get kinder in the mirror and in our minds. Then it can look like telling a friend, or five, or your whole following on social media about The Glitch. It may look like delving further into more learning around this subject. Or asking your HR, Inclusion or Wellbeing people at work to take a look at what we offer to help raise awareness. It can look like: throwing your scales away; buying clothes that fit; buying from companies who truly model diversity; avoiding fat talk among friends; finding non-image-based compliments for your friends; not being a sofa body critic or talking diets at home. It can be modelling better values for our kids, having real conversations with them and unpicking and de-coding our digital worlds with them. Or run petitions, complain about adverts, write to your MP, re-tweet sub-standard brand messaging (it really works), question our world and what it's showing us.

I really hope you've found this book valuable. Who can you pay it forward to? Who can you tag in a post about it?[5] Who can you share some of the parts that stay with you, next time they're body bashing or worse discriminating? Can you write a review and post it on your feed or Amazon or Good Reads to let others know?

Some will call me naïve, I'm sure, utopian, idealist. They will say, 'Darlin' that's not the way the world works', and to them I say, enough. This is *our* world. We can make it the world that we want, we just need to want… something else. To support something else, educate around a different conversation, create a different reality, emphasis on the real.

I am here standing on the shoulders of giants. Of Taryn Brumfitt (Embrace Documentary) and Elena Rossini (The Illusionists Documentary), of all the great academics out there researching this subject, Kim Chernin, Jean Kilbourne, Fiona Holland, Jessica Alleva, Phillipa Dietrichs, Shelly Grabe, Gemma López-Guimerà and spokespeople and supporters, Caryn Franklin, MP Mike Amesbury, Gok Wan, Rosie Nelon and the many influencers doing great work in this sphere, but I'm not standing, I'm crouching I'm reaching down to those who can make the next move, the next push, whether in your own lives or cultural moves that can shift this conversation on again. I can't stand until I am supporting you. So I need you to reach up and grab a hold in whatever way you can, even if it's just paying this book forward.

It's March 2021 and what a year it's been! Like my recovery, at the time, I had no idea where it would lead me, what positivity could possibly emerge from it, I just knew it would. And I know it now. (I'm not ashamed of how shmaltzy this has veered by the way.)

---

[5] You'll find example posts pinned to the top of my twitter feed and facebook group

There is so much negativity around at the moment. And I'm scared to try and counteract it because I know what hardships people are going through, I don't want to be insensitive to that at all. However like my cancer, in the thick of it, I couldn't tell the bounty that would come of it. Covid has given many people and the world at large, a rest. An opportunity to pause and regroup. To consider if we're going in the right direction. Are we aligned with our purpose? How can we improve our world? Equally as Dawn French has pointed out, this will prove a time of astonishing creativity. It has certainly been less commercial and it has given us a taste of less pressure. I've heard many of my friends rejoicing in a simpler life. It's made us realise all the stuff that we don't need, that we can live without. That we took for granted or that we'll be soooo grateful for, when we get them back.

But also, many of us might have spent longer looking at ourselves on Zoom or Teams calls, many of us have spent even longer on social media. Our bodies might have changed, our minds and feelings might have changed. But it might have also given us time to reflect, what do I really want, when no one is looking?

It's been poop so let's put that fertiliser to some good use! When we build the world again, let's do all the right things. Recovery was a challenge and this too has been too much in a lot of ways. This ten days alone we've had International Women's Day, the Megan/Oprah interview, we've learnt of Sarah Everard's tragic murder, eight are left dead in an Asian attack in Atlanta and there has been a lot of conversation.

We've watched Piers Morgan have a hissy fit. We've seen mental health and suicide be trivialised and as women we've felt the outrage that we all have this extra layer of fear in walking the streets.

I've learnt through a powerfully tearful TEDx talk that campaigner Gina Martin has been slut-shamed and has received so much vile online abuse[155] Why is this still happening? More technology running amok with no safety net[6]

Besides Gina Martin's success in criminalising up-skirting, a successful campaign by Nyome Nicholas-Williams, who took on Instagram and won, when they kept censoring her large black body in the way they didn't with white ones and Marcus Rashford's *Free School Meals Campaign,* there's still more we can do. In my echo chamber there's a lot of: 'Look, here I am again, it's me!' or the same shared memes. And I know, we're all busy. But here's a question, how is anything going to improve for us or future generations if we don't make the time? Prioritise it even. Could we align activism with our power, purpose and self-care and make space for it in our lives, even if it's just donating our time to a cause, signing a petition, even just engaging and commenting / supporting the posts of those activists you know – that helps because it means more people will see them. Because change would be good for all of us. And just because you can see someone else doing it, doesn't mean (a) it's taken care of or (b) they don't need your help. Hands down every activist is exhausted. Not by the work, by the continual drive to cut through the noise and get people to engage or rather disengage from the unreal world they're bug-eyed over.

What happened to activism? To feminism? To what we value, think, hold dear? To making a difference in the world. I remember a few years back, writing a feature about how I felt done-over by

---

6 We talk about 'breaking the internet'. In truth, nothing will break the internet. Unlike the B&Q fan that has just been recalled by mass email for being unsafe and not fit for purpose, the internet it seems has few limits for unsafe repercussions and no recourse. It's not really early days any more, so we can't blame that - this needs work.

feminism. Is this what they were all fighting for? In the 60s? Surely not, we've got half way there, the worst of both worlds – higher mortgages now everyone is working. overworked, underpaid, free and unvalued labour at home. I've provided almost full time childcare and haphazard cleaning while flexing my work around it, saving us multiple £1000s a year, for 13 years! It has been a compromise. I'm not saying my husband undervalued it. *I* did – financially, not emotionally; I would do it all again. It's just, nobody warned me. At school I was told that I could do anything, be anything. Have it all.

And we stopped being active on the issues that most affect us; probably because we're flipping exhausted! We only have the capacity to zone out. Annnnd still with the pay gap for those of us who make the humans, those mothers who chose to compromise themselves the other way. Meanwhile feeds are full of, 'Looky here I am in my fly joggers, feeling cute, might delete later'. What's happened to us? Do we mean to be doing this? You know the power this tech gives us right?

Racism, sexism, male violence have always been here, but we've had all these lockdown feelings because a lot of us are not (as usual) busy doing other things so we can really pay attention. Many of us, I know not all of us, but many currently have the time and the opportunity to feel and heal. To educate and explain, which I really hope helps us to emerge from this time stronger, more compassionate, with more understanding, more inclusion, more accountability into just basically a better world.

Sorry, that was a lot… again.

I was showering the other day, shaving my legs. You know… they're actually not that big. It made me reflect on my body and its performance.

I don't need it to sell bikinis or music or movies… I need it to live my life, do my work and support my family and friends and for that… it does it - and much more - beautifully.

I'll leave you with this quote from Elena Rossini's critically acclaimed The Illusionists:

'Across the world there are almost three billion people with an internet connection, 70% of them are online every day… This has the potential to be an almighty digital army that could be mobilised for change. Challenging the status quo, creating healthy media – taking on powerful corporations that profit from our insecurities.'[156]

'Only those who attempt the absurd, achieve the impossible'
Albert Einstein

Encore:

Conversations That *Probably* Will Never Happen (Probably)

Gabrielle's consciousness floated for minutes before it folded itself into coherent thoughts that could be classed as waking up. The usual, Who am I? Where am I? What's going on in my life? thoughts flitted on by. Growing awareness ratchetted up some tension. She found herself in the shower. Hot cloth face cleanser, colour grip shampoo, sink deep conditioner, pearl exfoliator, moisture rose foam, aloe razor, body wrap renew-you body gel.

Hair wrap, towel-dry, body butter to prolong the fake tan, foot cream. Teeth brushed, eyebrows plucked, eye gel, moisture lock serum, day cream, deodorant. Underwear, shapewear, boob boost, tan tights, pencil skirt, pretty blouse, necklace, earrings. Curl boost, barrel brush, hair dryer, curling tongs, fix spray. Rosacea calm, primer, foundation, concealer, eye base, illuminator, shadow blend, eye liner, draw eyebrows back in, brush brows and assess false eyelashes, contour, blusher, lip liner, lipstick, fragrance. Stilettoes. Hand cream.

- 16. The number of beauty products the 'average woman' uses a day.[157]

- £570 is a woman's average annual beauty product spend.[158]

- 55 minutes per day - time spent or a total of 14 full days a year.[159]

But Gabrielle would not thank you for assuming she was 'average'.

At the office Gabrielle brews a cup of herbal tea and opens her green juice.

'Hey!' calls Jenna from the storeroom. 'Did you see the latest deals coming in for the Seychelles? They're looking really good.'

'I'll take a look' Gabrielle replied. 'Mmmm, they're really pushing it this year, the operator might want to send someone on a discovery visit!' Gabrielle walked over to the shelves of holiday brochures and picked one up with a hammock, sugar white sand and curacao blue waters on the cover. She opened it and her attention fell into the paradise inside.

The door opened, bell tinkled and a commotion bustled through the door. Gabrielle turned and faltered slightly on her heels, she continued to struggle to stand still. Her mouth gawped. Eventually she, 'Erm, good… morning? Ah is this some kind of joke?'

The alicorns looked at each other.

'Joke?'

'Nope, no joke.'

'And you are… just a pair of fancy dress winged unicorns popping down the shops are you?' Gabrielle asked.

'Why does everyone keep saying 'fancy dress' to us Jumanka?'

'I don't know Sharapai, we're not even *wearing* dresses.'

Jenna appears from the storeroom and instantly drops a handful of post-it notes. 'What the…?'

Gabrielle says 'Ummm…'

Jumanka pitches in 'We're looking for flights.'

'Or a package deal,' continues Sharapai.

'We want to go to The Beautiful Place' Jumanka says.

'OK' replies Jenna, 'Well we have so many beautiful places we can… offer.'

'Yes' Gabrielle shakes her head and blinks into action 'The Seychelles might be just what you're looking for.' She steps forwards and offers the brochure in her hands, flicks through a few pages. 'Is this the sort of thing you're looking for?'

'Erm, not… exactly.' Sharapai replies.

'How about Australia?' Jenna offers and brings forth another brochure. The alicorns turn their long faces to the new offering. Gabrielle notices that their rainbow manes are pretty matted with bits of leaves and what look like tiny pumice stones embedded in them.

The winged unicorns make polite sounds about the brochures but then Sharapai hoofs around in her handbag and pulls out some folded papers (don't ask how).

'This, this is what we're looking for. We want to go to the place where these people are.'

'Yeah,' agreed Jumanka 'is it some kind of theme park or something?'

Jenna unfolded the thin papers.

'You see, this is what we came for. And we can't find it anywhere. The transmissions we get at home.'

'Home?'

'Yeah on Jupiter.'

'Jupiter!'

'Well yeah. The transmissions are full of these humans. These humans driving cars, these humans eating food, kissing humans, even these humans, happy at the dentist!' Jumanka was incredulous.

'Or when they're on their reproductive cycles' offered Sharapai.

'Yeah they're the ones I want to meet the most.'

'They're so happy ALL. THE. TIME! I really want to know their secret.'

'So you're… aliens?' asked Jenna.

'I mean, well, yeah, I guess to *you* we are.' Sharapai explained as Jenna passed some of the clippings to Gabrielle.

'Ah remember Sharapai, this is a patriarchal society, like, that was obvious even from home.'

'That's right,' Sharapai was laughing now 'they think all aliens are little green…'

'Men…' said Gabrielle looking confused '…not'

'Majestic unicorns?' Jenna chipped in.

'Alicorns actually' corrected Jumanka 'On account of the wings' and she flapped them for emphasis, upsetting rows of brochures 'Oh… sorry.'

Gabrielle was gazing at the visitors' greying gnarly hoofs, wondering why they didn't file and buff them, slick a brush of varnish over them. They'd look so much better. She brought her attention back to the clippings. They were adverts and blogs, editorials, pictures of people and the alicorns were right. They were all extatically smiling, even this lady selling washing up liquid. Yeay for chores!

'The thing is girls,' the alicorns shared a quizzical look, 'we sell beautiful places. Experiences'

'Right,' nodded Jumanka.

'There isn't a destination where these people are.' Gabrielle explained.

'But how can that be?' asked Sharapai 'We've travelled many miles to get here, we've been sent by officials to garner knowledge on happiness. So far… it's been…'

'Well it's been a little disappointing.' Jumanka finished.

'I mean, no offence' chipped in Sharapai 'You're just not… this,' and she hoofed at the paper. 'They're so glowy and smiley and you seem a little… sad.'

'Yeah, a lot of people seem sad,' agreed Jumanka.

Gabrielle looked at the papers again and sighed.

'Listen,' said Jenna, 'if you're looking to study happiness, you can't start with these. They're not… real.'

'WHAT!' the alicorns said in unison.

'You're telling us, there's nowhere on this planet that we can find these humans, how is that even possible?' Jumanka was understandably unsettled.

'I mean they *are* human, people, they just don't normally look like this.'.

'No they're more… normal in real life."

'You mean like you two?'

Gabrielle and Jenna exchanged a look.

'Yeah'

'Well no, maybe, not exactly. These people are chosen because they are… different than the rest of us.'

'So they do exist'

'Well yeah,'

'But no.'

'They don't look exactly like this.'

'They've had a lot of work done to look like this.'

'So what you're saying is it is possible to see humans like this, if they've had the work done.'

'Well no. Some of the work is done using technology. So imperfections have been removed and that glowy feel is added. Look.'

Jenna takes out her phone and takes a photo of the alicorns. She then puts a filter on the picture and shows them.

'Whoaaaa! That's amazing!'

'Look at my eyes, they're like flying saucers!'

'And we're glowy! Not so sharp, more fuzzy.'

'But the main thing is, if you were to meet these people, they're just normal people. Real lives, real problems. What you see of them is them telling a story, playing a role. Being a version of themselves that is…'

'Fake?' alicorn unison again.

'So *not* happy then' concluded Jumanka.

'… No. Sorry.'

'That makes me so… unhappy!' exclaimed Jumanka 'I can't be like them. Not ever?'

'Not ever,' sighed Jenna.

'Well, you could spend some time getting close… apart from you're a… what are you again?' asked Gabrielle.

'Alicorns.'

Gabrielle strode over to her bag and rummaged around inside. She found a wide toothed comb.

She returned to the alicorns and began the task of untangling their manes. Sharapai first. Twigs and space dust started to litter the carpet.

'Does this make you happy?' Sharapai asked.

'It's more just what we do. But yeah, I suppose on some level, it makes me happy. You'll have to see when it's finished, if it makes you happy.'

'So where do we go?' asked Jumanka 'To study happiness?'

'Erm… '

'Well…'

After some thought Jenna offered 'Inside yourself, find out who you are and appreciate what makes you happy and… do that.'

IN MEMORY OF:

Dad – Dr Wilf Howe
Aunty – Aileen Surtees
Trista, Cathy, Claire

Dr Kim Chernin who passed away with Covid, December 2020

A Soundtrack to Ditch the Glitch

- Paloma Faith - Never Tear Us Apart
- Alicia Keys and Brandi Carlile - A Beautiful Noise
- Ella Henderson - Glorious
- Meaghan Trainor - It's All About That Bass
- Lizzo - Good As Hell
- Mumford and Sons – Awake My Soul
- Jess Glynn – Thursday
- Paloma Faith – Make Your Own Kind of Music
- Joe Cocker - Have a Little Faith in Me
- Keala Settle and The Greatest Showman Ensemble - This is Me
- David Guetta ft. Sia – Titanium
- Rihaana - Diamonds
- Katy Perry – Roar
- Andra Day - Rise Up
- Robbie Williams – I Love my Life
- Florence and the Machine - Dog Days are Over

Support Links

For immediate help in an emergency:

- Call 999
- Go to your nearest A&E department

In a crisis and in need of talking to someone

- Call NHS 111 (for when you are in need of help but are not in immediate danger
- Contact your GP for an emergency appointment
- Samaritans – www.samaritans.org - 116 123
- Rethink Mental Illness - www.rethink.org National Advice Service: 0300 5000 927
- PAPYRUS UK - the national charity dedicated to the prevention of young suicide- www.papyrus-uk.org Helpline: 0800 068 4141
- Talk Club - a talking movement for men - www.wetalkclub.com/
- For a counsellor near you https://www.bacp.co.uk/
- Beat – The UK's Eating Disorder Charity - www.beateatingdisorders.org.uk – 0808 801 0677
- Breast Cancer Now – www.breastcancernow.org – Talk to a breast care nurse – 0808 800 6000

  Macmillan Cancer Support - www.macmillan.org.uk – 0808 808 00 00
- The Nipple Innovation Project – www.nippletattoos.co.uk charity@nippletattoos.co.uk
- You in Mind – Finding local Cheshire-based support - www.youinmind.org

- The Miscarriage Association – Helpline – 01924 200 799 www.miscarriageassociation.org.uk
- Hub of Hope – www.hubofhope.co.uk
- Mind - www.mind.org.uk - 0300 123 3393
- The Mental Health Foundation - www.mentalhealth.org.uk Specialising in policy development and research, and not able to advise people directly on their personal circumstances.
- Help Guide - www.helpguide.org/articles/anxiety/cutting-and-self-harm.htm (they give good info on how to stop self harm etc.)
- Young Minds - www.youngminds.org.uk/find-help/feelings-and-symptoms/self-harm/

Young Minds also Provides free, 24/7 text support for young people across the UK experiencing a mental health crisis. Helpline: 0808 802 5544 Text: YM to 85258

- Campaign Against Living Miserably - www.thecalmzone.net, Helpline: 0800 58 58 58, Webchat: www.thecalmzone.net/help/webchat/
- Sane - Support Forum: www.sane.org.uk, Call 07984 967 708

For the Kids

If you're keen to start the conversation with your little ones about how amazing and powerful our bodies are, grab a copy of Don't Go Knocking at the Circus Door.

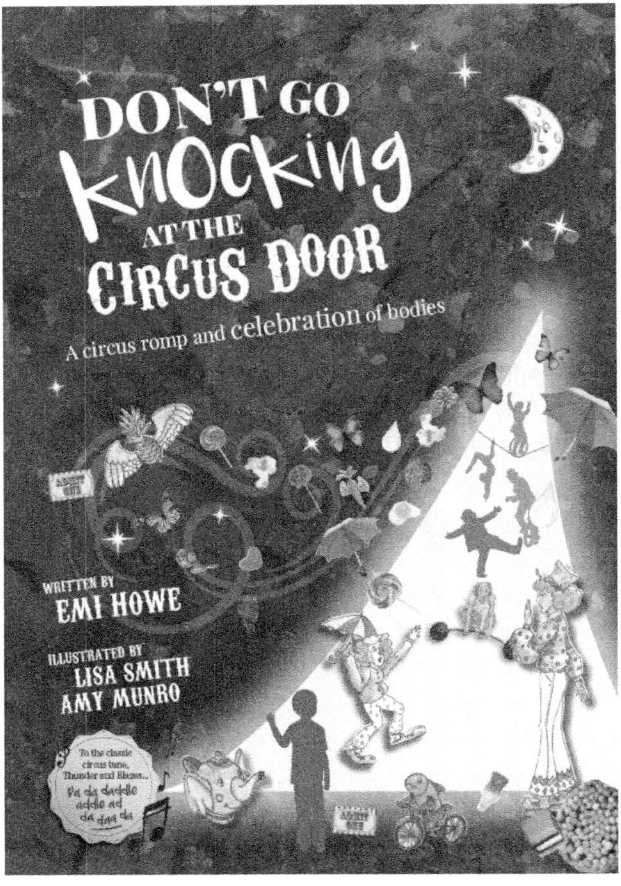

A show-stopping, sing-a-long storybook with activities to support learning. Available at: www.circus-door.co.uk and Amazon

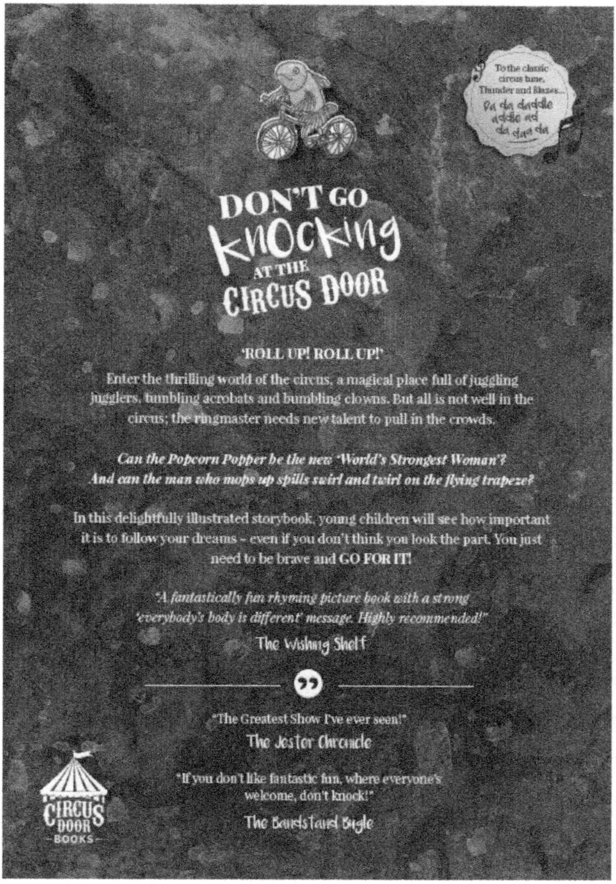

About the Author

Also by Emi Howe

Children's picture book celebrating bodies:
Don't Go Knocking on the Circus Door

Since her cancer diagnosis, Emi Howe has been on a mission to uncover everything she can to support her real body values and has reaped the benefits beyond measure. Emi is a writer, researcher, campaigner and advocate of body reality. A member of The Speaker's Collective, Corporate Advisor - instrumental in M&S's 2019 diverse lingerie branding and a school and workplace educator. She has created body-real resources for groups of all ages. Emi is a multi-nominated body therapist and is raising two body-savvy kids.
Emi has been published on/in: The Mighty, Huffington Post, Sky, Company, and writes / collates the blog BodEquality.com. Emi appeared in: Land Rover's #hybernot campaign; the 2017 Breast Cancer Awareness campaign for M&S and on Loose Women talking about body confidence.

'I have an incessant need to understand behaviour. It fascinates me because it opens a door to change, awareness, progress. This book is the most useful thing I could do with that part of me, and I'm grateful to have been able to do it. Truly, thank you for reading.'

Emi xx

Contact

If you have questions, please direct them to the BodEquality facebook group forum for an engaged chat: www.facebook.com/groups/BodEquality

To book Emi as a speaker please contact:
The Speakers Collective
www.speakerscollective.org – info@speakerscollective.org

Instagram: @BodEquality @TheCancerNude

You can visit www.bodequality.com to download a work pack

To bring BodEquality into your workplace, please email: info@BodEquality.com

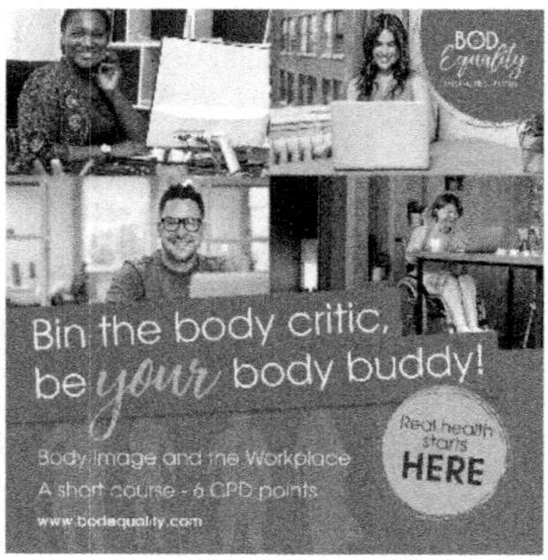

Acknowledgements

For Liz, my consultant and surgeon, Pauline, my health care worker, Jo my additional surgeon, Lisa, my breast care nurse, Ron, my chemo nurse and Lucy from Skinflicted and Stacie Rae from A.R.T. for my nipples and the Nipple Innovation Project – I don't know how I can better say it…just thank you. For photographer Jaine Briscoe Price and her loving and continual support of me and our work together @thecancernude on Instagram.

So many people for their support and encouragement over the years. My girls who all bring love and gorgeous friendship but also: my cousin Alli Saunders, wing woman Leana Hughes and her long-time support of this work – literally hours of listening to and considering with me, Amy Munro for impeccable design every time and everything you've contributed to this project over the years - truly thank you, Lisa Smith for artistry, Lynn Portis for encouragement and consideration of the topic, Charlotte Willis for guaranteed sensible conversation and being a human Google, Rowena Richardson for copy editing and sound advice, Katie North, Carolyn Stratton, Kathryn Usher, Adele Fieldz, Claire Swift, Rachel Jackson, Teena George, Karen Blundell-Servern, Sally Chappell. For Bex Gardner – and her unerring positivity and encouragement. For our friends The Joneses, The Whelans, The Murrays, The Allens. For Diane and the Tea Rooms Ladies, Andrea (Roomie), Erica, Sonia, Sarah W, Sarah T, Sharoonie, Georgina, Jo (and Rose), Julia, Louise, Jayne, especially Kate and also especially Becci (for TEDx).

For my mentors Atif Ahmed, Dianne Walker, Alan McKie, Stephanie Rosilio, also the support of Patricia Keating, Nicola Ellis, Natasha Blandthorn, UK Fast and TechManchester. For Ivan the Great (film maker), for my marketing intern and all-round Gift from the Universe, Nadia Deuskar. To Jo Emmerson, Marsha McAdam, Jon Salmon, Laura Phelan, Dave Chawner, Tom Ryder, Stephen Bell, Peter Larkum, George Hodgson, Nicholas Jametta and the Speakers Collective; BodEquality contributors: Fiona Holland (and Aiden), Pavie Valsa, Sumayra Ahmad, Clara Holmes, Hope Virgo, Kirpal Bhogal, Jonathan Cann, James Makings, Jonathan Holbrook, Jsky, Gus Bhandal, Nyome Nicholas-Williams, Roger Sim, Sarah Johnson, Amanda Hampton, Nicci Take – The Corporate Drag Queen.

For support along the way thanks to Michael Hogan, Annie Walling, Jen and Kat on the Naked Podcast, to TEDx folks Catherine Sandland, Samantha Newey, Ashley Costello.

Also Joshua Rowley of Rubenstein Library, Duke University, Rachel Peru, David Fadd, Stevie Blaine – A.K.A. bopo.boy, Andrea Boutin, Joules von Hep, Beth Willis Haviland, Melissa Gale, Emma Lanford, Mousse T, Emma Rees, Naomi Wolf, Kate Blakemore, Rachel Walker, Kathryn Leighton, Elena Rossini, Jessica Alleva, Jean Kilbourne, Phillipa Dietrichs, Christie Newman, Kate Fox, Shelly Grabe, Gemma López-Guimerà, Runa Uddin, Maria Katsarou, Mark Portis, Gareth Jackson (tech wizard), Phil Hughes, Todd.

To contributors: Caryn Franklin, M.G. Zimeta, Bev Carter, Leana Hughes, Gus Bhandal, Nick Butcher, Hannah Proverbs-Howe, Sarah Hollebon, Harpreet Chana, Ben Akers, John Barry, Chevy Rough, Jessica Joan Richards, Kerry Rycroft, Steve Loft, Molly Forbes.

To Steve Rowe, Dominic Fry and Carmel McQuaid, Meaghan Annear, Heather McLeod (HAM) and my gorgeous co-Ambassadors: Katie, Helen, Laura, Heather, Hayley, Lesley. To Linda Johansson, hair and make-up and for teaching me about eyebrows. Also Lou Box, hair and make-up, Rachell Smith, photographer, Kara Kyne – Stylist, Liz Unna - Director.

Thank you Cressida – The Book Analyst, Lisa Navarro of Navarro Law Consultancy. Thank you to first readers: Jennifer Lloyd, Melanie Spratley, Sheila Gee.

To Keryn Legg, Sarah Pearson and Nurit Pinko for being the keepers of my body while you help it relax, let go or repair.

For our families (including The Duchess), for making us who we are today and supporting this work with childcare! And especially Mum, Alli and Phil for their contributions. But mostly, to my incredible husband and kids, thank you for giving me the time. And for being my greatest gift. Aren't we so lucky!

References

[1] Kesses, E. (2016) *Why we need to change the way we market to women*, Campaign, www.campaignlive.co.uk https://www.campaignlive.co.uk/article/why-need-change-market-women/1417401

[2] Markham, A. (2010) *What Does Advertising Do? When you don't pay attention to ads, they affect you,* https://www.psychologytoday.com/gb/blog/ulterior-motives/201008/what-does-advertising-do#:~:text=These%20results%20suggest%20that%20the,other%20things%20that%20you%20like.&text=The%20feelings%20we%20have%20are,likely%20to%20turn%20out%20well.

[3] Markham, A. (2010) *What Does Advertising Do? When you don't pay attention to ads, they affect you,* https://www.psychologytoday.com/gb/blog/ulterior-motives/201008/what-does-advertising-do#:~:text=These%20results%20suggest%20that%20the,other%20things%20that%20you%20like.&text=The%20feelings%20we%20have%20are,likely%20to%20turn%20out%20well.

[4] Markham, A. (2010) *What Does Advertising Do? When you don't pay attention to ads, they affect you,* https://www.psychologytoday.com/gb/blog/ulterior-motives/201008/what-does-advertising-do#:~:text=These%20results%20suggest%20that%20the,other%20things%20that%20you%20like.&text=The%20feelings%20we%20have%20are,likely%20to%20turn%20out%20well.

[5] Crawford R. *Healthism and the Medicalization of Everyday Life.* International Journal of Health Services. 1980;10(3):365-388. doi:10.2190/3H2H-3XJN-3KAY-G9NY

[6] Kilbourn, J. (1995) *Slim Hopes: Advertising and the Obsession with Thinness*, Media Education Foundation

[7] Fox, K. (1997) Mirror, Mirror*, A summary of research findings on body image*, Motives: why we look in the mirror. Social Issues Research Centre, http://www.sirc.org/publik/mirror.html

[8]Gilday, K. (1990) *The Famine Within*, National Film Board of Cancada

[9] Newman, Christy. (2007*). Reader Letters to Women's Health Magazines: Inscribing the "will to health*". Feminist Media Studies. 7. 155-170. 10.1080/14680770701287027.

[10] Hawkins, N. (2014) *Battling our Bodies: Understanding and Overcoming our Negative Body* IMAGe – Centre for Change - https://centerforchange.com/battling-bodies-understanding-overcoming-negative-body-images/

[11] Gordon, A. (2020) *What we don't talk about when we talk about fat*, Beacon Press Audio

[12] Yeboah, S. (2020) *Fattily Ever After – A Fat, Black Girls Guide to Living Life Unapologetically*, Hardie Grant Books, Bolinda Audio

[13] Newman, Christy. (2007). *Reader Letters to Women's Health Magazines: Inscribing the "will to health"*. Feminist Media Studies. 7. 155-170. 10.1080/14680770701287027.

[14] Meyers, G.J. (2010*) The Tudors: The Complete Story of England's Most Notorious Dynasty.* Delacourte Press.

[15] Royal Museums Greenwich, (Accessed 08 Dec 2020) *Little known or unknown facts regarding Queen Elizabeth 1's Death* - https://www.rmg.co.uk/discover/explore/little-known-or-unknown-facts-regarding-queen-elizabeth-is-death

[16] Collishaw, M. (13 November 2018*) Behind the Mask of Youth* – Royal Museums Greenwich - https://www.rmg.co.uk/discover/behind-the-scenes/blog/behind-mask-youth#:~:text=The%20Mask%20of%20Youth%20was,to%20emphasise%20her%20youthful%20appearance.&text=Paintings%20that%20didn't%20comply%20with%20the%20ideal%20appearance%20were%20destroyed.

[17] Goodman, R. (2013) *How to be a Victorian*. Viking publishing - P67

[18] Gunderman, R., (9th June 2015*) The manipulation of the American mind: Edward Bernays and the birth of public relations* in www.theconversation.com https://theconversation.com/the-manipulation-of-the-american-mind-edward-bernays-and-the-birth-of-public-relations-44393

[19] Digital Deli Online (N.D.) *Kelloggs* http://digitaldeliftp.com/LookAround/advertspot_kelloggs.htm

[20] Mayyasi, A (9th May 2016) *Pricenomics – How breakfast became a thing* https://priceonomics.com/how-breakfast-became-a-thing/

[21] 500px (N.D.) The Story Behind Jenifer in Paradise – The First Photoshop Image - https://iso.500px.com/the-story-behind-jennifer-in-paradise-the-first-photoshop-image/

[22] Burns, M. (20, Feb 2015) *Thomas Knoll: 4 things I've learned from developing the original Photoshop* – Digital Arts from IDG

[23] The Editors of Encyclopaedia Britannica (8th November 2019) *Adobe Photoshop* - https://www.britannica.com/technology/Adobe-Photoshop

[24] Merriam-Webster. (n.d.). Photoshop. *In Merriam-Webster.com dictionary.* Retrieved March 12, 2021, from https://www.merriam-webster.com/dictionary/photoshop

[25] A. H. Maslow (1943) A Theory of Human Motivation
Originally Published in Psychological Review, 50, 370-396. Accessed from http://www.researchhistory.org/2012/06/16/maslows-hierarchy-of-needs/?print=1

[26] Brumfitt, T. (2016) Embrace Documentary - www.bodyimagemovement.com/embrace/embracethedocumentary/

[27] Bryson, B. (2019) *The Body: A Guide for Occupants* - Penguin Random House.

[28] Gordon, A. (2020) *What we don't talk about when we talk about fat*, Beacon Press Audio

[29] O'Rahilly, S. (2020) (Cambridge) 1: *The Causes of Obesity: Why isn't everybody fat?* https://www.youtube.com/watch?v=zMjS_X5Hk7Y

[30] Warner, A. (2019) – *The Truth about Fat – Why Obesity is not that Simple* – Oneworld Publications

[31] Robinson, S. (July 18th 2019) *This Woman Shared What Her Sled Dog Team Taught Her About Body Positivity, And It's Perfect*, Buzz Feed, https://www.buzzfeed.com/sydrobinson1/dogs-body-positivity

[32] Bartlett, D (1st July 2013) *The Reason 90% of Diets end in Failure* in The Huffington Post https://www.huffingtonpost.co.uk/daniel-bartlett/weight-loss-diet-failure_b_3185060.html

[33] Friedman, J. (Oct, 2014) *20 years of Leptin: Leptin at 20 – An overview in the journal of Endochrinology* - Volume 223: Issue 1 https://joe.bioscientifica.com/view/journals/joe/223/1/T1.xml

[34] Niedhammer, F (2020) 45 Minute Gentle Yoga for Beginners Breathe and Flow Yoga

[35] Karolinska Institutet. (2014, September 2). *Childhood trauma could lead to adult obesity*. ScienceDaily. Retrieved January 24, 2021 from www.sciencedaily.com/releases/2014/09/140902092947.htm

[36] University of Southern California (June 28, 2017) *The Link Between Childhood Trauma and Obesity*, Suzanne Doworak-Peck school of Social Work, https://dworakpeck.usc.edu/blog/the-link-between-childhood-trauma-and-obesity#:~:text=Obesity%20as%20a%20Defense%20Mechanism,developing%20obesity%20as%20an%20adult

[37] Mayor, S. (2017) Socioeconomic disadvantage is linked to obesity across generations, UK study finds

BMJ 356:j163 www.bmj.com/content/356/bmj.j163.full

[38] Maclellan, L. (2019) New Research *Examines the Treacherous Experience of Being "Fat"*

AT Work – Quartz at Work - https://qz.com/work/1702660/

[39] Gordon, A. (2020) *What we don't talk about when we talk about fat*, Beacon Press Audio

[40] Cotter, A. (2020) *Olive, Mabel and Me – Life and Adventures with two very good dogs* – Black and White Publishing

[41] We Are Tilt (2021) The Benefits of Flexible Thinking – BBC Ideas - Made in partnership with the Open University

[42] Fox, K. (2004) *Watching the English – The Hidden Rules of English Behaviour* Hodder

[43] Muhlheim, L. (2021) *Eating Disorder and Suicide Risk*, Very Well Mind, https://www.verywellmind.com/eating-disorders-suicide-4174291

[44] Akers, B. (2019) Steve Documentary - **www.stevedocumentary.com**

[45] Eccleston, C. (2019) I Love the Bones of You - My Father and the Making of Me, Simon and Schuster

[46] Haggerty, J. (2017) *Why You Gain Belly Fat After Menopause (and why it's ok)* https://www.jessihaggerty.com/blog/why-you-gain-belly-fat-after-menopause-and-why-its-ok?fbclid=IwAR1gPDvIHMflpoOSEkv5leh3_tKN1goVQjwiN6RZWZP_h0r35nf8XXBEvTM

[47] Brown, H. (2015*) Medical Examiner, The Weight of the Evidence - It's time to stop telling fat people to become* THIN. https://slate.com/technology/2015/03/diets-do-not-work-the-thin-evidence-that-losing-weight-makes-you-healthier.html

[48] Mumsnet (2018) I hate the body positive movement - www.mumsnet.com/Talk/am_i_being_unreasonable/3248015-to-hate-the-body-positive-movement

[49] Yeboah, S. (2020) *Fattily Ever After – A Fat, Black Girls Guide to Living Life Unapologetically*, Hardie Grant Books, Bolinda Audio

[50] Cordon, J. (2019) *James Corden Responds To Bill Maher's Fat Shaming Take,* twitter.com/latelateshow/status/1172571955314094080

[51] Grabe, S. et al. (2008) *The Role of the Media in Body Image Concerns Among Women: A Meta-Analysis of Experimental and Correlational Studies* in American Psychological Association 2008 Vol 134, No 3, 460-476

[52] Sánchez, David & Neumark-Sztainer, Dianne & López-Guimerà, Gemma. (2012). Integrated prevention of obesity and eating disorders: Barriers, developments and opportunities. Public health nutrition. 15. 1-15. 10.1017/S1368980012000705.

[53] Gordon, A. (2020) *What we don't talk about when we talk about fat*, Beacon Press Audio

[54] Luppino FS, de Wit LM, Bouvy PF, et al. *Overweight, Obesity, and Depression: A*

Systematic Review and Meta-analysis of Longitudinal Studies. Arch Gen Psychiatry. 2010;67(3):220–229. doi:10.1001/archgenpsychiatry.2010.2

[55] Goldberg, C. (2019) *Study: Bias Drops Dramatically For Sexual Orientation And Race — But Not Weight* https://www.wbur.org/commonhealth/2019/01/11/implicit-bias-gay-black-weigh

[56] Oakes, K. (2019) *The Complicated Truth About Social Media and Body Image* BBC Future, https://www.bbc.com/future/article/20190311-how-social-media-affects-body-image

[57] Chernin, K. (2013) *Our Hungry Selves: Women, Eating and Identity*, Psychotherapy.net, LLC https://www.psychotherapy.net/article/women-eating-disorders-kim-chernin

[58] Mussett, S. (N.D.) *Simone de Beauvoir* (1908—1986), https://iep.utm.edu/beauvoir/

[59] Kesses, E. (2016) *Why we need to change the way we market to women*, Campaign, https://www.campaignlive.co.uk/article/why-need-change-market-women/1417401

[60] goodreads (2012) Thomas S. Monson Quotes - www.goodreads.com/quotes/495000-we-can-t-direct-the-wind-but-we-can-adjust-the

[61] Gray, C. (2017) *The Unexpected Joy of Being Sober*, Aster, An Hachette UK Company, P169

[62] Hay, L. L. (1984) *You Can Heal Your Life*, Hay House P49

[63] Yeboah, S. (2020) *Fattily Ever After – A Fat, Black Girl Guide to Living Life Unapologetically*, Hardie Grant Books, Bolinda Audio

[64] The Human Experience Podcast (n.d.) EPISODE 63 – *Gabor Maté M.D. – When the Body Says No,* https://thehumanxp.com/episode-63-gabor/

[65] Bryson, B. (2019) *The Body, A Guide for Occupants*, Penguin, Random House

[66] Alleva, J. M et al. (2018) *A randomised -controlled trial investigating potential underlying mechanisms of a functionality-based approach to improving women's body image. (Using British Women)* From The Department of Clinical Psychological Science, Maastricht University, Maastricht, The Netherlands, Centre for Appearance Research, University of the West of England, Bristol, UK, Jean Golding Institute, University of Bristol, Bristol, UK. In journal: Body Image – 25 (2018) 85 – 96

[67] PACEY, (2016*) Children as Young as Three Unhappy with their Bodies.* https://www.pacey.org.uk/news-and-views/news/archive/2016-news/august-2016/children-as-young-as-3-unhappy-with-their-bodies/

[68] Balantekin, K., Birch, L. Savage, J. (2015) *Patterns of Weight Control Behavior Among 15 year old Girls* - Intl Journal of Eating Disorders - https://www.ncbi.nlm.nih.gov/pmc/articles/PMC4542016/

[69] Judith, B (2016) *Body Image 'A Problem for Boys', Says Advertising Think Tank,* BBC News Credos, 2016 - https://www.bbc.co.uk/news/education-37010205

[70] Halliwell, E, Diedrichs, P. C, Orbach, S. (2014*) - Costing the invisible: A review of the evidence examining the links between body image, aspirations, education and workplace confidence.* https://uwe-repository.worktribe.com/output/806655

[71] Warner, A. (2019) – *The Truth about Fat – Why Obesity is not that Simple* – Oneworld Publications

[72] NHS (2018) *BMI Healthy Weight Calculator, Healthy Weight,* https://www.nhs.uk/live-well/healthy-weight/bmi-calculator/

[73] Warner, A. (2019) – *The Truth about Fat – Why Obesity is not that Simple* – Oneworld Publications P77

[74] Barber, N. (2010) *So You Think That Losing Weight Will Make You Healthy?* Think Again. Psychology Today, https://www.psychologytoday.com/us/blog/the-human-beast/201007/so-you-think-losing-weight-will-make-you-healthy-think-again

[75] Warner, A. (2019) – *The Truth about Fat – Why Obesity is not that Simple* – Oneworld Publications P77

[76] Fox, K. (2004) *Watching the English – The Hidden Rules of English Behaviour,* Hodder and Stoughton, p 125

[77] Hosie, R., (16th March 2017) *How Women's Bodies Have Changed since 1967* – The Independent Newspaper, Indy/Life section https://www.independent.co.uk/life-style/health-and-families/womens-body-changes-1957-self-image-fashion-weight-health-sizes-positive-a7633036.html

[78] Strong-Duncan. M. (2018) I Believe 'Stranger Things' Made A Risky Casting Choice, Here's Why, Odyssey, **https://www.theodysseyonline.com/stranger-things-recast-**

[79] Jessyas (2017) Is Natalia Dyer from Stranger Things anorexic? – Reddit - https://www.reddit.com/r/StrangerThings/comments/4tf495/is_natalia_dyer_from_stranger_things_anorexic/

[80] Auerback, A. (2019*) Flex, The Modern Woman's Handbook, HQ*, p61

[81] Clifton, R. (2020) *Love your Imposter – Be your best self, flaws and all.* Kogan Page Ltd

[82] Simpson, P. (2017) *Reaping the Benefits of a Focus on Wellbeing -Special Report* – Health Sector, Financial Times - Reaping the benefits of a focus on wellbeing | Financial

Times (ft.com)

[83] The Chartered Institute of Personnel and Development (March 2020) *Wellbeing at Work, Survey Report*, Health and well-being at work | CIPD

[84] Fielding, H. (1996) *Bridget Jones Diary* – Picador

[85] Winman, S. (2015) *A Year of Marvellous Ways,* Headline Publishing Group

[86] Knowles, B. (2019) HOMECOMING, Netflix, Parkwood Entertainment

[87] Robinson, E. (12, May, 2017) *Female Mannequins aren't just Skinny they're Emaciated* – The Guardian.

[88] Piepenbring, D. (2016*) The Case of the Shrinking Mannequins, and other news*, The Paris Review, https://www.theparisreview.org/blog/2016/09/13/case-shrinking-mannequins-news/

[89] Zimeta, M.G. (2016*) In John Lewis*, London Review of Books, https://www.lrb.co.uk/blog/2016/september/in-john-lewis

[90] ASA (3rd June 2014) *Advertising Standards Authority: Every UK ad a responsible ad* on YouTube www.youtube.com/watch?v=0xjTJoLklvs

[91] Advertising Standards Authority (17th July 2017) *Social Responsibility: Body Image.* https://www.asa.org.uk/advice-online/social-responsibility-body-image.html

[92] ASA (3rd June 2014) Advertising Standards Authority: Every UK ad a responsible ad on YouTube www.youtube.com/watch?v=0xjTJoLklvs

[93] Petitions: UK Government and Parliament (8th July 2018) *Require in law that branding/ads must show a variety of real body shapes* https://petition.parliament.uk/archived/petitions/208103

[94] Clarkeson, E. (2017) Can I Speak to Someone in Charge - Simon and Schuster

[95] Nelson, R. (n.d. c.2016) *Create a Law to Protect Models from being Pressured to Lose Weight* – Change.org - https://www.change.org/p/cj-dinenage-create-a-law-to-protect-models-from-getting-dangerously-skinny-lfw-modelslaw

[96] Guilbault, L. Garced, K. Szmydke, P. (22, Dec 2015) *Fashion Execs react to tough French laws on thing models.* Women's Wear Daily - https://wwd.com/fashion-news/fashion-features/fashion-reaction-french-law-skinny-models-10302035/

[97] Beat. (2018) *The UK's leading charity supporting those effected by eating disorders* https://www.beateatingdisorders.org.uk/

[98] Guilbault, L. Garced, K. Szmydke, P. (22, Dec 2015) *Fashion Execs react to tough French laws on thing models.* Women's Wear Daily - https://wwd.com/fashion-news/fashion-features/fashion-reaction-french-law-skinny-models-10302035/

[99] Metro (3 Nov 2009) Gok: Teach body confidence to kids – www.metro.co.uk/2009/11/03/gok-teach-body-confidence-to-kids-531483/

[100] The Telegraph (4 Nov 2009) Gok Wan – Calls on Teenagers to be given body confidence lessons - www.telegraph.co.uk/news/health/news/6496879/Gok-Wan-calls-on-teenagers-to-be-given-body-confidence-lessons.html

[101] Media Smart (2021) Media Smart – Home – www.mediasmart.uk.com

[102] ASA (2021) About the ASA and CAP - www.asa.org.uk/about-asa-and-cap/about-regulation/about-the-asa-and-cap.html

[103] BEAT (9/1/2017) *Beat welcomes Theresa May's comments, BEAT* eating Disorder Charity https://www.beateatingdisorders.org.uk/news/beat-welcomes-theresa-mays-comments

[104] BEAT (15/11/2017) *Three-and-a-half-year delay for eating disorder treatment worsens illness and cost to the NHS*, BEAT eating Disorder Charity https://www.beateatingdisorders.org.uk/news/three-half-year-delay-eating-disorder-treatment

[105] Owens, M. (9/8/2019) *What really is the cost of obesity to the NHS.* Adam Smith Institute. https://www.adamsmith.org/blog/what-really-is-the-cost-of-obesity-to-the-nhs

[106] Stice, E., and Shaw, H.E. (Nov 2002) *Role of body dissatisfaction in the onset and maintenance of eating pathology: A synthesis of research findings*, Journal of psychosomatic research, 53(5). 985-993.

[107] Grabe, S. et al. (2008) *The Role of the Media in Body Image Concerns Among Women: A Meta-Analysis of Experimental and Correlational Studies* in American Psychological Association 2008 Vol 134, No 3, 460-476

[108] Thompson et al. in Calgero, R & Thompson J.K. (2007) *The Impact of Western Beauty Ideals on the Lives of Women: A sociocultural perspective*, The body beautiful, 259-298

[109] Alleva, J. M et al. (2018*) A randomised -controlled trial investigating potential underlying mechanisms of a functionality-based approach to improving women's body image. (Using British Women)* From The Department of Clinical Psychological Science, Maastricht University, Maastricht, The Netherlands, Centre for Appearance Research, University of the West of England, Bristol, UK, Jean Golding Institute, University of Bristol, Bristol, UK. In Journal: Body Image – 25 (2018) 85 – 96

[110] López-Guimerà et al. (2010*) Influence of Mass Media on Body Image and Eating-Disordered Attitudes and Behaviours in Females: A Review of Effects and Processes.* In Media Psychology, 13: 387-416, Taylor and Francis Group, LLC.

[111] Grabe, S. et al. (2008*) The Role of the Media in Body Image Concerns Among Women: A Meta-Analysis of Experimental and Correlational Studies* in American Psychological

Association 2008 Vol 134, No 3, 460-476

112 Striegel-Moore, R. H., & Bulik, C. M. (2007). *Risk Factors for Eating Disorders.* American Psychologist.

113 Be Real (Feb 2018) *In Your Face: A report investigating young people's experiences of appearance-based bullying. Body Confidence for everyone* In partnership with YMCA and Dove

114 ASA (3rd June 2014) Advertising Standards Authority: Every UK ad a responsible ad
on YouTube www.youtube.com/watch?v=0xjTJoLklvs

115 Heller, S. (Mar. 30, 2018) *People can't get enough of ASOS' new swimsuit model, and say it's game-changing to see their own bodies represented*, Business Insider.

116 Grabe, S. et al. (2008) *The Role of the Media in Body Image Concerns Among Women: A Meta-Analysis of Experimental and Correlational Studies* in American Psychological Association 2008 Vol 134, No 3, 460-476

117 Irving, L.M., & Berel, S. (2001) *Comparison of media literacy programs to strengthen college women's resistance to media images.* Psychology of Women, 6.

118 McVey , G. L., & Davis, R. (2002) *A programme to promote positive body image: A 1-year follow-up evaluation.* Journal of Early Adolesence, 22.

119 ASA (N.D.) *Senior Management* - https://www.asa.org.uk/about-asa-and-cap/people/asa-senior-management.html

120 CAP Committees, Panels and Executive: https://www.asa.org.uk/about-asa-and-cap/people/cap-panels-and-committees.html#CAP

121 Stice, E., and Shaw, H.E. (Nov 2002) *Role of body dissatisfaction in the onset and maintenance of eating pathology: A synthesis of research findings,* Journal of psychosomatic research, 53(5). 985-993.

122 Grabe, S. et al. (2008) *The Role of the Media in Body Image Concerns Among Women: A Meta-Analysis of Experimental and Correlational Studies* in American Psychological Association 2008 Vol 134, No 3, 460-476

123 Grabe, S. et al. (2008) *The Role of the Media in Body Image Concerns Among Women: A Meta-Analysis of Experimental and Correlational Studies* in American Psychological Association 2008 Vol 134, No 3, 460-476

124 Grabe, S. et al. (2008) *The Role of the Media in Body Image Concerns Among Women: A Meta-Analysis of Experimental and Correlational Studies* in American Psychological Association 2008 Vol 134, No 3, 460-476

125 Greenberg, B. S. et al. (2009) *A Portrait of Food and Drink in commercial TV series.*

Health Communication, 24

[126] UKEssays. (November 2018). *Mass Media Effects On A Girls Body Image Media Essay.* Retrieved from https://www.ukessays.com/essays/media/mass-media-effects-on-a-girls-body-image-media-essay.php?vref=1

[127] López-Guimerà et al. (2010*) Influence of Mass Media on Body Image and Eating-Disordered Attitudes and Behaviours in Females: A Review of Effects and Processes.* In Media Psychology, 13: 387-416, Taylor and Francis Group, LLC.

[128] Grabe, S. et al. (2008) *The Role of the Media in Body Image Concerns Among Women: A Meta-Analysis of Experimental and Correlational Studies* in American Psychological Association 2008 Vol 134, No 3, 460-476

[129] Be Real (Feb 2018*) In Your Face: A report investigating young people's experiences of appearance-based bullying. Body Confidence for everyone* In partnership with YMCA and Dove

[130] Grabe, S. et al. (2008) *The Role of the Media in Body Image Concerns Among Women: A Meta-Analysis of Experimental and Correlational Studies* in American Psychological Association 2008 Vol 134, No 3, 460-476

[131] British Youth Council (2017) *A Body Confident Future* – Youth Select Committee.

[132] CAP (2018) Gender Stereotyping – A Consultation on CAP and BCAP's proposal for a rule and guidance to address the use of gender stereotypes in advertising – Committee of Advertising Practice – Pg 4

[133] ASA (3rd June 2014) Advertising Standards Authority: Every UK ad a responsible ad
on YouTube www.youtube.com/watch?v=0xjTJoLklvs

[134] CAP (2018) Gender Stereotyping – A Consultation on CAP and BCAP's proposal for a rule and guidance to address the use of gender stereotypes in advertising – Committee of Advertising Practice – Pg 7

[135] British Youth Council - (2017) *A Body Confident Future* - Youth Select Committee

[136] CAP/BCAP (2018*) Gender stereotypes in advertising CAP and BCAP's evaluation of responses,* https://www.asa.org.uk/uploads/assets/uploaded/03e2fb9c-f878-4c65-81344257b667d1ab.pdf

[137] CAP/BCAP (2018) *Gender stereotypes in advertising CAP and BCAP's evaluation of responses,* https://www.asa.org.uk/uploads/assets/uploaded/03e2fb9c-f878-4c65-81344257b667d1ab.pdf

[138] CAP/BCAP (2018) *Gender stereotypes in advertising CAP and BCAP's evaluation of responses,* https://www.asa.org.uk/uploads/assets/uploaded/03e2fb9c-f878-4c65-81344257b667d1ab.pdf

[139] CAP/BCAP (2018) *Gender stereotypes in advertising CAP and BCAP's evaluation of responses,* https://www.asa.org.uk/uploads/assets/uploaded/03e2fb9c-f878-4c65-81344257b667d1ab.pdf

[140] CAP/BCAP (2018) *Gender stereotypes in advertising CAP and BCAP's evaluation of responses,* https://www.asa.org.uk/uploads/assets/uploaded/03e2fb9c-f878-4c65-81344257b667d1ab.pdf

[141] ASA (2017) *Depictions, Perceptions and Harm, A Report on Gender Stereotypes in Advertising,* www.asa.org.uk/resource/depictions-perceptions-and-harm.html

[142] Martin, G. (2019) Be The Change - Sphere

[143] Tech Manchester (Accessed Dec 2020) *About Tech Manchester* - https://techmanchester.co.uk/about

[144] Clifton, R. (2020) *Love your Imposter – Be your best self, flaws and all.* Kogan Page Ltd.

[145] Warner, A. (2019) – *The Truth about Fat – Why Obesity is not that Simple* – Oneworld Publications.

[146] BBC News (27,7,2020) *Coronavirus is a 'real moment for action' on obesity* www.bbc.co.uk/news/av/health-53551703

[147] Udemy (2018) Udemy in Depth – Workplace Distraction Report https://research.udemy.com/research_report/udemy-depth-2018-workplace-distraction-report/

[148] Simpson, P. (2017) *Reaping the Benefits of a Focus on Wellbeing -Special Report* – Health Sector, Financial Times - Reaping the benefits of a focus on wellbeing | Financial Times (ft.com)

[149] The Chartered Institute of Personnel and Development (March 2020) *Wellbeing at Work, Survey Report,* Health and well-being at work | CIPD

[150] Chernin, K. (2013) *Our Hungry Selves: Women, Eating and Identity,* Psychotherapy.net, LLC www.psychotherapy.net/article/women-eating-disorders-kim-chernin

[151] BBC News (2020) *Lizzo sparks body debate with 10-day smoothie diet* , Entertainment and Arts, www.bbc.co.uk/news/entertainment-arts-55315796

[152] Chernin, K. (2013) *Our Hungry Selves: Women, Eating and Identity,* Psychotherapy.net, LLC www.psychotherapy.net/article/women-eating-disorders-kim-chernin

[153] Warner, A. (2019) – *The Truth about Fat – Why Obesity is not that Simple* – Oneworld Publications.

[154] UK Parliament (2020 *Changing the perfect picture: what can be done about poor body image?* https://committees.parliament.uk/committee/328/women-and-equalities-committee/news/119399/changing-the-perfect-picture-what-can-be-done-about-

poor-body-image/

[155] Martin, G. (2020) They told me to change my clothes. I changed the law instead. TEDx Warwick https://www.youtube.com/watch?v=_K_n-x-W7pY

[156] Rossini, E. (2016) *The Illusionists*, https://theillusionists.org/

[157] Lifestyle (2017) *The average woman used 16 beauty products a day* – The Telegraph - https://www.telegraph.co.uk/beauty/face/essential-skincare-makeup-products-use-everyday/

[158] Buglass, L. (2019) *This is how much the average woman spends on skincare a year* , Woman and Home, www.womanandhome.com/beauty/beauty-news/average-woman-spends-skincare-321315/#:~:text=This%20is%20how%20much%20the%20average%20woman%20spends%20on%20skincare%20a%20year&text=To%20celebrate%20the%20launch%20of,570%20on%20skincare%20each%20year.

[159] Thapoung, K. (2014) *You'll Be Shocked By How Long Women Spend on Their Hair and Makeup Each Day,* Women's Health Mag - https://www.womenshealthmag.com/beauty/a19954807/womens-beauty-routine/

Printed in Great Britain
by Amazon

59071980R00244